Current Approaches

Obsessive Compulsive Disorder

Edited by
S A Montgomery, W K Goodman and Nicola Goeting

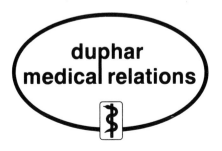

duphar
medical relations

First published 1990

ISBN 1-870678-21-4

Printed in Great Britain by Ashford Colour Press, Gosport, Hampshire.

CONTENTS

CHAIRMAN'S INTRODUCTION

Obsessive compulsive disorder is an illness that is now receiving a great deal of attention both in the scientific literature and in the media. The reasons for this increase in interest are made clear in this collection of papers from a symposium held in London on 6 April 1990.

It is now known that the disorder is more common than was initially assumed, and, as a chronic and disabling illness, it represents substantial morbidity. At the same time many more sufferers are coming forward for care now that new effective treatments are becoming available which are also less time consuming than earlier treatments offered.

We need to ensure that treatments are effective and the discussion of the measures and methods required to establish efficacy are very welcome. The relative roles of drug or behavioural treatments or possible combinations is an important issue and both approaches are well represented in this volume.

There is increasing evidence that the serotonergic system plays an important part in obsessive compulsive disorder, a view which was stimulated by the quite specific therapeutic response to potent serotonergic drugs and supported by the studies of neuroendocrine response to serotonergic probes. The nature of the response to these serotonergic drugs, which differs markedly from the response expected in depression or anxiety, has added weight to the argument that OCD is an illness which should be separated from the anxiety disorders. The diagnostic distinctiveness of OCD is strengthened by genetic studies and by the fascinating link with the tics and movements seen in Gilles de Tourette syndrome.

It remains for us to thank Professor Isaac Marks, who chaired the morning session, the individual authors for their contributions and Dr Nicola Goeting of Duphar for her courtesy and forebearance in helping to speed the production of this book.

STUART MONTGOMERY
WAYNE GOODMAN

IS OBSESSIVE COMPULSIVE DISORDER DIAGNOSTICALLY INDEPENDENT OF BOTH ANXIETY AND DEPRESSION?

Stuart A Montgomery

St Mary's Hospital Medical School, London

Obsessive compulsive disorder (OCD) is an odd and quite distinctive illness. The condition is found to be rather common in epidemiological studies, with a life time prevalence of 2.5‰ reported in the large Epidemiological Catchment Study (ECA) carried out in the United States.[1] The nature of the illness, with its characteristic obsessions and rituals, makes it easy for the sufferers to recognise the disorder in themselves but in spite of this only a small proportion attend for treatment. Only 26% of those diagnosed as suffering from OCD in the ECA study had attended for treatment in a six month period, compared with 38% for major depression, and 50% for panic disorder. This low attendance figure for a distinctive, chronic and fluctuating illness with high stability of diagnosis might well reflect, among other factors, the dissatisfaction of sufferers with the treatment offered. The ECA study was carried out in the US before the introduction of any 5-HT uptake inhibitors, now the treatment of choice in Europe, and in that country. It would be interesting to see whether these rates of attendance change now that more effective treatment is generally available and OCD is recognised as a treatment indication in the US. This is not however the only explanation. Sufferers from OCD will often recognise that they have unwanted thoughts or behaviours that may be disabling but fail to perceive these as a disorder for which a remedy might be sought. One of the tasks facing us therefore is to *teach* both doctors and sufferers to recognise the disorder for which treatment is relatively easily available.

The separation of OCD from the anxiety disorders

OCD is currently classified under the anxiety disorders in both DSMIIIR and ICD diagnostic schemes. The rationale for this has not been properly established and there is an increasing body of data suggesting that this is inappropriate. The symptom complexes seen in OCD are quite distinctive and readily separate OCD from other related conditions, a separation that is supported by other fundamental differences.

Sufferers from OCD mostly have a long, chronic, fluctuating course of the same identifiable illness, Rasmussen and Tsuang[2] reported that in the overwhelming majority of their patients a chronic waxing and waning course was observed. The persistence and high stability of the diagnosis contrasts with anxiety states which tend to change their nature over time and become depression at later follow up. The stability of the condition is a good guide to the separate identity of the disorder. There are moreover interesting differences in the appearance of the illness. The sex distribution of OCD is roughly equal[1] which is quite different from anxiety states where females outnumber males by 2:1. Different age of onset might also indicate separate disorders. In the ECA study the age of onset of anxiety states was much earlier than OCD while in this study it was closer to depression.[3]

The treatment response data in OCD is quite different from that seen in anxiety states. Conventional anxiolytics such as benzodiazepine appear ineffective as do those other drugs widely used in anxiety states such as MAOIs and neuroleptics. Conventional tricyclic antidepressants such as amitriptyline, nortriptyline, imipramine and desipramine which are widely used in anxiety appear to be ineffective in OCD in so far as they have been tested. The response to placebo is strikingly different being high in anxiety states and very low or absent in OCD. OCD contains within its psychopathology a number of anxiety symptoms and the failure of the studies of anxiolytics to demonstrate efficacy suggests that OCD does not properly belong within the anxiety disorders. By contrast clomipramine is effective in treating the anxiety symptoms of OCD which suggests that these anxiety features are an integral part of the illness rather than a secondary feature.

Is OCD part of depression?

A proportion of patients with OCD develop quite profound depressive symptomatology, and the controversy as to whether these depressive symptoms are integral to the OCD or a separate secondary disorder is unresolved. Symptoms of OCD and depression commonly occur together in the same patient; for example in the ECA study approximately one third of patients with a diagnosis of OCD also fulfilled DSMIII criteria for major depression. OCD and depression both tend to appear in the same families suggesting an association between the two illnesses, though the nature of the possible link is unclear.

Obsessional symptoms are sometimes seen in clearly defined major depression; but these are seen to be related to depressive symptomatology, obsessional thoughts of guilt for example. In many OCD patients, however, depressive episodes supervene upon a background of longstanding obsessive compulsive disorder. This has led some investigators to attempt to separate the diagnosis of depression and OCD on the basis of precedence so that OCD can only be diagnosed if it occurred first. The evidence from the treatment studies of OCD, however, favours the recognition of OCD as a distinct illness which has associated depressive and anxiety symptoms, and which appear to respond as part of the OCD.

2

Difference in response between OCD and depression

OCD resembles depression in that the only drugs that have been found to be effective in OCD are drugs which have also been shown to be effective in depression. OCD, however, appears to respond only to serotonergic drugs and not to other antidepressants, which makes it a more specific illness than depression.[4] Clomipramine, fluvoxamine and, to a lesser extent, mianserin, for which placebo controlled efficacy has been shown in OCD, are all drugs with potent serotonergic properties, the first two being potent 5-HT uptake inhibitors, and mianserin being a 5-HT1, 5-HT2 and 5-HT3 receptor antagonist.

The depressive symptoms in OCD appear to respond in parallel with the improvement in the OCD as is seen in the reports of Flament et al,[5] Perse et al,[6] Cottraux et al,[7] and Goodman et al.[8] Although two early studies did not find an association between response of depressive and obsessional symptoms[9,10] these were limited by being very small. It is interesting that in the study of Goodman et al[8] the response of the depressive symptoms was unlike that seen in depression, being rapid, with a significant difference from placebo appearing at two weeks. This time course of response that is consistently seen in OCD is unlike that seen in depression and indicates that the depressive symptoms are integral to the OCD.

Low placebo response in OCD

Another feature which helps us to differentiate OCD from depression is the poor response to placebo seen with OCD. For example, in the study of Montgomery,[11] placebo was associated with a response rate of some 5%, whereas the response to clomipramine was 65%. A low placebo response rate was also seen in both of the large multicentre studies in which a highly significant advantage for clomipramine was confirmed.[12] The ability for the clinical studies to establish efficacy, even though the number of patients included was quite small in some of them, may be due, in part, to the consistently low or absent placebo response, which is seen whether or not there was concomitant depression. A placebo response rate of 30% or greater is expected in depression, and it is not unusual for a rate of nearer 50% to be reported. In OCD the depressive symptoms do not appear to respond to placebo. Furthermore although the data are rather sparse and not entirely consistent it seems that the depressive symptoms associated with OCD do not appear to respond to antidepressants which are ineffective in OCD. Any effect of nonserotonergic antidepressants is weak. The general lack of response of depressive and obsessional symptoms to placebo or reference antidepressants suggests that depressive symptoms are integral to the OCD and respond as part of the treatment of the OCD.

Early response to 5-HT uptake inhibitors in OCD.

The response to 5-HT uptake inhibitors in OCD was seen as a significant difference from placebo in the early study of Montgomery[11] at weeks 1, 3, and 4. This early response was confirmed in the two large multicentre studies of de-Veaugh Geiss *et al*[12] who reported a significant difference from placebo from one to two weeks. The response in the 5-HT uptake inhibitor treated groups in these studies appears linear, with an incremental response seen over many weeks. This early response was also reported by Goodman *et al*[8] with fluvoxamine.

A response so early in treatment is not expected in depression treated with 5-HT uptake inhibitors or for that matter any antidepressants. A significant difference from placebo cannot be reliably shown in depression until four weeks of treatment. In this respect OCD differs markedly from depression and it is suggested that the mechanism of action of 5-HT uptake inhibitors, thought to involve secondary adaptive receptor changes which produce the anti-depressant effect, is different in OCD where the effect is more direct.

The separation of OCD from major depression

The fact that the depressive symptoms, and for that matter the anxiety symptoms, fail to respond to antidepressants that do not have potent serotonergic properties, the relative lack of a placebo response rate which would be expected to a substantial extent in depression, and the very early onset of a significant response compared with placebo all mark out OCD as a disorder which is separate from major depression.

The other evidence which should be considered is the different sex distribution between the illnesses. In depression the distribution is two females to one male and OCD is quite different in being more evenly distributed between the sexes. The time course of the illness is also rather different from depression, which is seen as an episodic illness, the episodes being separated by long periods in remission. OCD in contrast is perceived as a chronic disorder with a fluctuating waxing and waning course.

Factors affecting response rates

The response rates in the different studies are seen to vary from one study to another, and there are several possible explanations for this phenomenon. Firstly the sensitivity of the scales used to measure change varies and one explanation advanced for the varying response rates is that a higher response rate may be detected by the more sensitive scales such as the obsessional scale constructed from the CPRS. However this is unlikely to be the complete or only explanation and other factors may be expected to contribute.

Ritualisers versus ruminators

One way of subdividing OCD is by the presence of predominant obsessional thoughts in the ruminators or of predominant rituals in the ritualisers. The ECA study suggests that ruminators are slightly more common in the community whereas in many treatment studies ritualisers predominate.

The selection of patients for different studies may vary, depending on the source of referrals and the nature of the practice of different clinics. It is possible, for example, that OCD clinics with a behaviourial orientation preferentially attract ritualisers. The inclusion of a high proportion of ritualisers, who may have a different response compared with ruminators, might lead to a different in response rates being registered in some clinics. This attractive theory is however not supported by the data.

5-HT uptake inhibitors have been found to be effective compared with placebo in behaviour therapy oriented centres with a high proportion of ritualisers[7,13] as well as in centres including a high proportion of ruminators.[11] Furthermore it appears that clomipramine is effective in treating both rituals and obsessional thoughts in the predominantly ritualiser group.[13] It would appear that 5-HT uptake inhibitors are effective in treating both sets of symptom-complexes and selection bias on this basis is not critical for response.

Presence of concomitant depression

A similar argument has been advanced that a better response to 5-HT uptake inhibitors is seen in OCD with concomitant depression than in pure OCD. This theory is also not borne out by the treatment response data which suggest that the response rates are similar in pure OCD and OCD with concomitant depression. It appears that the depressive symptoms are integral to OCD and are likely to respond in parallel with the obsessional symptoms.

OCD with tics or movement disorders

Another factor which is more likely to be important is the inclusion of OCD with concomitant movement disorders. In OCD there is an increased chance of an occurrence of Gilles de la Tourette Syndrome (GTS) and some centres have higher rates of concomitant GTS than others. From our experience OCD with GTS does not respond well to 5-HT uptake inhibitors, and we have been excluding these patients from our studies. The high response rate reported in the study of Montgomery[11] at 4 weeks, may partly reflect the enhanced efficacy in the pure group of OCD without concomitant movement disorders. It would be interesting to examine the data of those studies which have included both OCD with and without GTS, to see whether there is an improved overall response rate in the pure group. Goodman[14] suggests that this appears to be the case in his data set and recommends the use of concomitant neuroleptics with 5-HT uptake inhibitors to treat those with the overlapping syndromes of OCD together with GTS.

CONCLUSION

There is reasonable evidence that OCD is a stable disorder which should be viewed as diagnostically separate. The grounds for regarding OCD as part of the anxiety disorders are more historical than supported by data. OCD has a different sex distribution as well as different course and outcome. The response to treatment is different from both depression and anxiety disorders with a unique and particular response to serotonergic drugs and virtually no response to placebo. The depressive symptoms in OCD do not appear, as far as we can tell, to respond well to conventional antidepressants whereas they do respond to 5-HT uptake inhibitors. The disorder is in many ways unique and is recognised as a separate treatment indication in the U.S. For the time being it should also be thought of as a separate diagnosis and attempts should be made to encourage those who suffer from its long term personal and social damage to recognise that treatment is at hand.

REFERENCES

1 Karno M, Golding J, Sorenson S et al. The Epidemiology of Obsessive Compulsion Disorder in Five US Communities. Arch Gen Psychiatry 1988;49:1094–1099.

2 Rasmussen S A and Tsuang M T. Clinical characteristics and family history in DSMIII obsessive disorder. Am J Psychiatry 1986;143:317–322.

3 Burke J D, Regier D A, Christie K A. Epidemiology of Depression: recent findings from the NIMH epidermiologic catchment area programme. In: Depression and Anxiety eds. J A Swinkels, W Blijleven: Medidact Houten, 1988.

4 Montgomery S A, Fineberg N, Montgomery D B. The efficacy of serotonergic drugs in OCD – power calculations compared with placebo. This issue.

5 Flament M, Rapoport J, Berg C et al. Clomipramine Treatment of Childhood Obsessive Compulsive Disorder. Arch Gen Psychiatry 1985;42:977–983.

6 Perse T L, Greist J H, Jefferson J W et al. Fluvoxamine Treatment of Obsessive Compulsive Disorder. Am J Psychiatry 1987;144:1543–1548.

7 Cottraux J, Mollard E, Bouvard M et al. A controlled Study of fluvoxamine and exposure in obsessive compulsive disorders. Int Clin Psychopharmacol 1990;5:17–30.

8 Goodman W K, Price L H, Rasmussen S A et al. Efficacy of fluvoxamine in obsessive compulsive disorder. Arch Gen Psychiatry 1989;46:36–44.

9 Ananth J, Pecknold J L, Van den Steen N et al. Double blind comparative study of clomipramine and amitriptyline in obsession neurosis. Prog Neuro-psychopharmacol 1981;5:257–262.

10 Insel T R, Murphy D L, Cohen R M et al: Obsessive Compulsive Disorder – a double blind trial of clomipramine and clorgyline. Arch Gen Psychiatry 1983;40:605–612.

11 Montgomery S A. Clomipramine in obsessional neurosis: A placebo-controlled trial. Pharm Med 1980;1:(2), 189–192.

12 de Veaugh Geiss J, Landau P, Katz R. Treatment of obsessive compulsive disorder with clomipramine. Psychiatr Ann February 1989;19: (2), 97–101.

13 Marks I M, Stern R S, Mawson D, Cobb J and McDonald R. Clomipramine and exposure for obsessive compulsive rituals: I. Br J Psychiatry 1980;136:1–25.

14 Goodman this issue.

THE PREVALENCE OF OBSESSIVE COMPULSIVE DISORDER IN THE COMMUNITY

Paul Bebbington
Reader in Epidemiological and Social Psychiatry
Institute of Psychiatry, London

Obsessive compulsive disorder (OCD) seems to be one of the Cinderellas of psychiatric epidemiology. It has suffered from a concentration of interest on the big topics in the field – psychoses in general, schizophrenia, major affective disorder. Epidemiological surveys of psychiatric disorder often do not report findings relative to OCD, and even where they do they are presented as incidental. In other cases it is lumped together with neurosis NOS: those with a specific interest in OCD therefore have to search to discover what they want to know.

The central issue in epidemiological research is that of case finding. Before cases can be determined, there has to be an appropriate and useable definition of the disorder in question. One consequence of the limited epidemiological interest in OCD has been an insufficient attention to the job of defining it.

OCD in any case poses intrinsic problems in this respect. The first step must be an adequate description of key symptoms. Even today there is no consensus over exactly how this should be done, although their essential characteristics were recognised long ago. Moreover, in the author's experience, many clinicians find it difficult to grasp the essential attributes of these symptoms. Others report similar difficulties.[1] The basic ideas of compulsive intrusiveness and a sense of resistance are relatively easy to communicate, but applying these concepts to the mental experience of individual subjects requires the development of considerable clinical acumen.

Even if there were a reasonable consensus over the categorisation of obsessional and compulsive symptoms, difficulties would remain about how these should be used to define cases of OCD. A major problem is their frequent coexistence with other neurotic symptoms of depression and anxiety. In consequence, there is a need for rules determining when symptoms of OCD are merely part of a larger anxiety or depressive state, when they justify a separate diagnosis, and when they can be taken as sufficiently salient to make a primary diagnosis of OCD. As we shall see, solutions to this particular problem have been inadequate, and none has gained sufficient acceptance to dispel ambiguity from epidemiological studies.

Psychiatric community surveys now have a long history. The first attempts, in the early part of this century, were poorly resourced and based on methods of case finding with all the scientific precision of investigative journalism. Typically, the research team would steep themselves in a local community,

7

esablish rapport with local agencies and key people, and ask around for information about those deemed to suffer from nervous conditions.[2,3] The researchers might accept local opinion about the actual diagnoses, or they might interview those thought to suffer from mental disorders. In the latter case, diagnosis was based on the ordinary clinical practice of the investigator with no attempt at standardisation.

Cases of OCD were reported from studies using these primitive methods: so, for instance, Roth and Luton[2] found 5 cases of OCD in a Tennessee Community of 1721 souls (0.3%) and Brunetti[4] found a single case among 102 subjects in rural Vaucluse, France. Clearly little can be concluded, except to wonder if OCD is actually quite rare in non-referred populations.

A second generation of psychiatric community surveys are of even less relevance to our search. They followed the development of standardised instruments for screening American military populations for unspecified psychiatric disturbance during the war.[5] They permitted a division of the population into broad bands representing supposedly increasing levels of psychiatric impairment, but were incapable of providing any diagnostic information.[6,7]

The 'third generation' of psychiatric community surveys[8] can be seen as a reaction to this nonspecificity and the resumption of a positive view of diagnosis. They are based on structured, standardised diagnostic interviews linked to algorithms generating classifications according to internationally accepted schemes. They fall into two groups based on the 9th Edition of the Present State Examination (PSE) and on the Diagnostic Interview Schedule (DIS).

Those two interviews differ in philosophy and content. The PSE allows the interviewer considerable latitude in deciding whether symptoms defined in a glossary are evident in the individual case. The necessary standardisation is provided by training courses and the glossary, but relies considerably on the clinical judgement of the interviewer. The DIS in contrast is absolutely structured, in an attempt to eliminate the need for clinical judgement altogether, so that the instrument can be used by lay interviewers with little or no experience of psychiatry. This approach carries the risk of sacrificing validity on the altar of reliability.

The two instruments also serve different classification systems. The PSE is linked through the CATEGO program with the 9th Edition of the International Classification of Disease. CATEGO embodies explicitly hierarchical principles, so that if a higher order diagnosis is met, symptoms of lower order conditions are largely disregarded in the process of classification. This has a crucial bearing on the epidemiological study of OCD with this instrument. If syndromes of generalised or specific anxiety are present, they take precedence over the obsessional syndrome, and the case is allocated to a category of anxiety neurosis or phobic neurosis. Moreover, cases in general population surveys using the PSE are invariably reported in terms of another algorithm, the Index of Definition (ID).[9] This programme allocates each subject to one of eight levels denoting increasing confidence in the clinical value of the categories proved by the CATEGO program. Community surveys conventionally define cases as those with an ID level of 5 and above. Where obsessional symptoms occur in relative isolation, subjects are usually not deemed to be cases at all. The consequence is that no PSE survey, except that in Santander, has found any cases of obsessional neurosis in the population studied. Vazquez-Barquero and his colleagues[10] did find a single case of obsessional neurosis, a woman, giving a female prevalence of 0.16%. We must therefore turn to the DIS studies for information about OCD in the community.

The DIS provides the basis of classification in terms of the DSMIII, the Feighner criteria and the RDC. So far, reports have been a DSMIII catagories.

DSMIII criteria for OCD are set out in Table 1. Most clinicians would agree they make quite a lot of sense. However, the key issue of when obsessional symptoms are adequate to substantiate a diagnosis of obsessional neurosis rather than forming part of some other diagnosis remains.

TABLE 1
Diagnostic criteria for Obsessive Compulsive Disorder
A. Either obsessions or compulsions:
Obsessions: recurrent, persistent ideas, thoughts, images, or impulses that are ego-dystonic, i.e., they are not as voluntarily produced, but rather as thoughts that invade consciousness and are experienced as senseless or repugnant. Attempts are made to ignore or suppress them.

Compulsions: repetitive and seemingly purposeful behaviors that are performed according to certain rule or in a stereotyped fashion. The behavior is not an end in itself, but is designed to produce or prevent some future event or situation. However, either the activity is not connected in a realistic way with what it is designed to produce or prevent, or may be clearly excessive. The act is performed with a sense of subjective compulsion coupled with a desire to resist the compulsion (at least initially). The individual generally recognizes the sense-lessness of the behaviour (this may not be true for young children) and does not derive pleasure from carrying out the activity, although it provides a release of tension.

B. The obsessions or compulsions are a significant source of distress to the individual or interfere with social or role functioning.

C. Not due to another mental disorder, such as Tourette's Disorder, Schizophrenia, Major Depression, or Organic Mental Disorder.

Whatever the reservations about the quality of DIS data, the studies based on it form our only sizeable body of knowledge about OCD in the community. Nine such studies have now been reported.[11-22] The first five comprised the Epidemiologic Catchment Area studies carried out in separate areas of the US as part of an integrated programme of epidemiological research. All the surveys were very large. Apart from the Taiwan study, the results were extremely consistent.

OCD is only one of the many diagnostic categories afforded by the DIS, and has not been the focus of individual reports. Nevertheless, the studies provide data about several basic epidemiological concerns.

What can clinicians reasonably require of epidemiological studies of OCD? They might wish to know how many people suffer or are likely to suffer from the condition, whether it is commoner in certain groups, when it starts, how long it lasts, how it is related to other psychiatric conditions, and how many generally need treatment. Tentative answers to these questions are now available.

The standard values provided by the DIS are for six-month prevalence and lifetime prevalence. In the first instance, subjects contribute to prevalence if they have met case criteria at any time during the six months preceding interview. This measure gives a very rough idea of how many members of the community might be candidates for treatment. However, conditions picked up in this way can be acute or chronic: some may be self-limiting, and some may have improved by the time of assessment. Life time prevalence is based on subjects who at any time have met the criteria of case definition. It provides only a crude index of the likely burden of disorder over time, as it is affected by the age structure of the population: old populations will have moved further throught the period of risk.

Values for the prevalence of OCD are given in Table 2. The figures for Taiwan are uniformly much lower than those for the other sites (this is true of

Table 2. Prevalence of Obsessive-compulsive Disorder (%) DIS studies

	Six-month	Lifetime
ECA sites		
New Haven	1.5	2.7
Baltimore	2.1	3.1
St Louis	1.3	1.9
Piedmont	2.2	
Los Angeles	0.7	2.1
Other sites		
Edmonton	1.6	3.0
Puerto Rico	1.8	3.2
Taiwan		
Taipei	0.3	0.9
Small town	0.1	0.5
Rural	0.1	0.3
Christchurch	1.0	2.2

virtually all diagnoses – it is not clear whether it represents an anomaly of DIS usage in this study or whether the Chinese really suffer from very low rates of mental disorder). The rates for the remaining sites are really very consistent, ranging from 0.7% to 2.2% for six month prevalence, and from 1.9% to 3.2% for life time prevalence. There is a suggestion from Los Angeles that Hispanics may have lower rates of OCD than Anglo-Americans.[13,14] However, this does not tally with the findings from Puerto Rico.[16] Canino and her colleagues manipulated their data in an interesting way: they *added* questions to the DIS in the section covering OCD, and as a result the lifetime prevalence fell from 3.2% to 1.1%. No details of these additional questions are given, nor any rationale for the procedure, but this underlines the crucial effect that changing definitions has on case finding.

From these data it might be inferred that around half of all subjects who have experienced OCD remain cases in the period before interview, suggesting that the disorder is of some persistence. This is expressed more formally in data for Christchurch and Edmonton (Table 3): the 'one-year recovered' rate indicates the proportion of subjects who have been deemed cases of OCD, but have not met the criteria in the year preceding interview.

Table 3. One Year Recovered Rates of OCD

Edmonton	39%
Christchurch	50%

Table 4 presents the sex-ratio of prevalence of OCD. This ranges between equality and a ratio of 1 male case to 2.3 female cases for six month prevalence. The range for life time prevalence shows greater variability. Overall it may be concluded that OCD is somewhat but not strikingly commoner in women, with a ratio of perhaps 1.5 : 1.

Table 4. Sex Ratio of Prevalence of Obsessive-compulsive Disorder DIS studies (female : male)

	Six-month	Lifetime
ECA sites		
New Haven	1.9	1.6
Baltimore	1.2	1.3
St Louis	1.9	2.4
Los Angeles		
Hispanic	1.2	1.8
Other		1.2
Other sites		
Edmonton	1.0	1.1
Puerto Rico	1.8	0.9
Taiwan		
Taipei		1.3
Small town		1.9
Christchurch	2.3	3.4

11

Another issue of interest to epidemiologists is the way prevalence varies with age. Data available from the DIS studies are given in Table 5 for six month prevalence. The age bands are fairly broad, but in general the greatest prevalence seems to be in the age bands below 45. The results from Edmonton are provided in more detail (Figure 1). In males, there is a peak between 35 and 54, whereas in females the peak is clearly in those between 25 and 34. Obviously too much must not be made of these figures because they are based on relatively few cases, but in line with clinical experience it does appear as though OCD is a condition typically affecting those in middle adulthood.

Table 5. Six Month % Prevalence of OCD by Age – DIS Studies

	18-24	25-44	45-64	65+
ECA sites				
New Haven				
Males	0.9	1.3	0.4	1.2
Females	2.7	2.8	0.8	0.4
Baltimore				
Males	2.1	1.7	2.4	0.9
Females	2.6	3.1	1.3	1.2
St Louis				
Males	1.5	1.3	0.2	0.2
Females	2.8	1.5	1.3	1.3
Other sites				
Puerto Rico	0.6	1.7	3.1	
Christchurch	1.0	1.1	0.8	

Figure 1. Six month prevalence of OCD by age

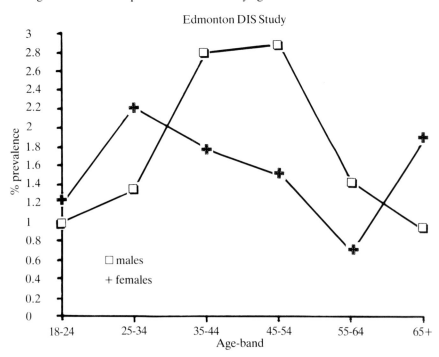

12

The variation by age of lifetime prevalence identifies potential problems with this index. If subjects were equally prone to OCD whatever their year of birth, a consistent increase of lifetime prevalence with age would be expected. However such an increase is only apparent in the findings from Puerto Rico (Table 6). In other centres, life time prevalence falls off with increasing age.[6]

Table 6. Lifetime % Prevalence of OCD by Age – DIS Studies

	18-24	25-44	45-64	65+
ECA sites				
New Haven	2.8	3.8	1.5	1.3
Baltimore	3.5	3.9	2.5	1.2
St Louis	2.2	2.4	1.4	1.1
Other sites				
Puerto Rico	1.9	2.5	5.3	
Christchurch	1.8	2.8	1.6	

This could indicate a cohort effect, that is, subjects with later birth dates may be increasingly prone to OCD. However, it is also apparent for the majority of other conditions. Either people are becoming more prone to psychiatric disorder in a completely non-specific way, or there is some other explanation. Perhaps the most likely possibility is that episodes are forgotten with the passage of time. In my view, cohort effects remain to be established.[23]

Because life time prevalence is distorted by the age structure of the population, measures which correct for this are of particular interest to geneticists. One such measure is lifetime morbid risk. Bland and his colleagues[17] provide estimates for this on the basis of their Edmonton data, with values of 5.4% for both men and women. In other words, the chance that someone will suffer OCD at some time during a life of normal length is 5.4%.

Data from the Edmondton study also give some idea of age of onset. This information is based on the appearance of the first symptoms of OCD, *not* on the date when subjects first met criteria for the diagnosis. Results must be interpreted accordingly. The mean age of first symptoms was 21.4 for males, 19.6 for females. The distribution of age of first symptoms is shown actuarily in figure 2, and confirms that the first manifestations are often very early.

Although the results reported from the community psychiatric surveys using the PSE do not illuminate the subject of OCD, such surveys have potential advantages for epidemiological work because they elicit symptoms of clinical significance. The studies to date have used the ninth edition of the PSE[24] which includes three items relating to OCD: obsessional checking and rituals, obsessional cleanliness, and obsessional ruminations. In the process of the CATEGO program, these items are first used to establish the syndrome ON (see Table 7). It is useful to study both the individual items and the amalgamation represented by the syndrome.

Table 7.

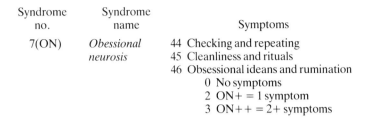

Syndrome no.	Syndrome name	Symptoms
7(ON)	*Obessional neurosis*	44 Checking and repeating
		45 Cleanliness and rituals
		46 Obsessional ideans and rumination
		0 No symptoms
		2 ON+ = 1 symptom
		3 ON++ = 2+ symptoms

Figure 2. Cumulative Distribution of Age of Onset

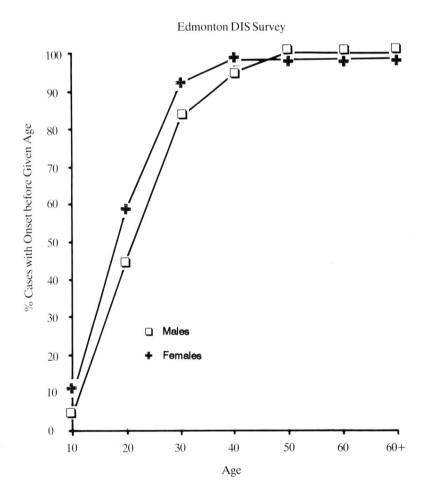

Edmonton DIS Survey

□ Males

+ Females

Age

% Cases with Onset before Given Age

14

The Camberwell Community Survey has been described in detail elsewhere.[25,26] It comprised a two-stage procedure whereby 800 subjects randomly selected from the population of Camberwell, South London, were interviewed by agency interviewers using a short version of the PSE. Further interviews with an MRC team were sought with all those rated 5 and over on the Index of Definition of the first interview. This second interview was based on the full version of the PSE and included the obsessional items. A random sample of those rated below ID level 5 were also re-interviewed, and a simple weighting procedure permitted the calculation of frequencies of symptoms in the original population.

Although the CATEGO program allocated no case to the Obsessional Neurosis *category*, the *syndrome* of Obsessional Neurosis was quite common, being picked up in 6.8% of males and 14.4% of females (10.8% overall). The frequency of the individual items is given in Table 8, and it is apparent that only obsessional checking is at all frequent.

Table 8. Weighted numbers and prevalence of selected symptoms in the Camberwell population

Symptom	Males		Females		Total
44 Checking and repeating	9	6.0	20	12.0	9.1
45 Cleanliness and rituals	0	0	5	3.0	1.6
46 Obsessional ideas and ruminations	2	1.6	1	0.3	0.9

It is possible to use data about symptoms to tell us more about the nature of obsessional disorders in the general population. It is of some interest to know how symptoms tend to cluster together. Some symptoms are 'powerful' in the sense that they are often associated with other neurotic symptoms. In other words having one of these key symptoms is predictive of a disorder of some severity. This issue can be explored by relating the presence of individual syndromes to overall PSE symptom scores. It is apparent from Figure 3 that the syndrome Obsessional Neurosis (ON) is associated with a lower total PSE score than the syndrome Situational Anxiety (SA). This suggests that subjects with obsessional symptoms lack any great tendency to suffer additionally, for instance, a wide range of anxiety symptoms. Specific phobias, as might be expected, are associated with even lower PSE scores. The relative dissociation of obsessional symptoms from other neurotic symptoms was corroborated by loglinear analysis of the contribution of obsessional symptoms and of general anxiety symptoms to total PSE score. This suggested that the contribution was essentially separate.

We are still some way from an estimate of the need for treatment for OCD in the general population. The threshold for recognising individual obsessional items is quite low in the PSE. Returning to check something more than three times, provided the other qualities of an obsessive symptom are present, is sufficient for a rating on item 44, although neither the subject nor the clinician would be likely to think the symptom worth treating.

A content analysis was carried out to illuminate the nature of the obsessive symptoms identified in the population at large. Of 36 subjects who were positively rated on obsessional items, eighteen exhibited longstanding checking at just over threshold level and essentially in isolation from other symptoms. One subject with mild compulsive handwashing also shared this sort of picture.

The remaining 17 subjects showed much more in the way of neurotic symptoms, but in every case but one the obsessional symptoms were minor additions to an overall pattern.

Altogether, only seven subjects were rated on compulsive washing and only three on obsessional ruminations. Only on three occasions in two subjects were obsessional items given a rating of '2', that is, severe. In the author's opinion, none of the mild symptoms required treatment; they caused little interference or distress, and subjects were content to live with them. So, for example, subject 521 was given to checking things that might be unsafe. He had even on occasions returned from work to check his heater, but not often. He was currently mildly depressed, and was placed at the threshold level 5 of the Index of Definition. He himself did not see the checking as a problem.

Only in one instance might a subject have benefited from specific treatment aimed at obsessional symptoms, although she did have a wide variety of other neurotic symptoms. Subject 585 had indeed suffered an episode of schizophrenia 4 years previously from which she had recovered. However, she was currently acutely depressed (ID7, PSE total score 31). She was a longstanding checker and handwasher, and was rated as severe on both items.

As a contrasting example, subject 851 was suffering from one of the most severe disorders we encountered in our community survey (ID7, PSE total score 47). She displayed a very severe mixed anxiety depressive state. She was a longstanding checker, but the symptom was only of mild intensity. The checking was the least of her problems, and was not felt to merit separate treatment.

The content analysis suggests that in a sample of 800 not otherwise remarkable for its vibrant mental health, one case alone was felt to merit treatment. A slightly larger number might have been found if we ourselves had interviewed the subjects at the first stage: however, I doubt this, and in any case it could make little difference to my opinion that very few members of the general population require treatment, even though minor obsessional symptoms are common. In consequence, my conclusions remain similar to those of Roth and Luton,[2] despite half a century of epidemiological progress.

REFERENCES

1 Mignolli, G., Faccincani, C., Burti, L., Gavioli, I., and Micciolo, R. Inter-rater reliability of PSE-9: an Italian study. *Social Psychiatry and Psychiatric Epidemiology* 1988; **23**:3-35.

2 Roth, W.F. and Luton, F.H. The mental health program in Tennessee. *American Journal of Psychiatry* 1942; **99**:662-675.

3 Brugger, C. Psychiatrische Ergebnisse einer Medizinischen, Anthropologischen und Soziologischen Befolkerungsuntersuchung. *Zeitschrift fur die Gesamte Neurologie und Psychiatrie* 1933; **146**:489-524.

4 Brunetti, P.M. Rural Vaucluse: Two surveys on the prevalence of mental disorders: summary of data. *Acta Psychiatrica Scandinavica, Suppl.* 1977; **263**:12-15.

5 Stouffer, S.A., Guttman, L., Suchman, E.A., Lazarsfeld, P.F., Star, S.A. and Clausen, J.A. Measurement and prediction. In: *Studies in Social Psychology in World War II, Vol. IV.* Princeton University Press, Princeton. 1950.

6 Srole, L., Langner, T., Michael, S.T., Opler, M.K. and Rennie, T.A.C. *Mental Health in the Metropolis.* New York: McGraw-Hill 1962.

7 Leighton, A.H. *The Character of Danger (Stirling County Study Vol.2).* New York, Basic Books. 1963.

8 Dohrenwend B.P. and Dohrenwend B.S. Perspectives on the past and future of psychiatric epidemiology. *American Journal of Public Health* 1982; **72**:1271-1279.

9 Wing, J.K., Mann, S.A., Leff, J.P. and Nixon, J.M. The concept of a case in psychiatric population surveys. *Psychological Medicine* 1978; **8**:203-217.

10 Vazquez-Barquero, J-L., Diez-Manrique, J.F., Pena, C., Aldana, J., Samaniego-Rodriguez, C., Menendez-Arango, J. and Mirapeix, C. A community mental health survey in Cantabria: a general description of morbidity. *Psychological Medicine* 1987; **17**:227-242.

11 Myers, J.K., Weissman, M.M., Tischler, G.L., Holzer, C.E., Leaf, P.J., Orvaschel, H., Anthony, J.C., Boyd, J.H., Burke, J.D., Kramer, M. and Stolzman, R. Six month prevalence of psychiatric disorders in three communities: 1980-1982. *Archives of General Psychiatry* 1984; **41**:959-67.

12 Robins, L.N., Helzer, J.E., Weissman, M.M., Orvaschel, H., Gruenberg, E., Burke, J.D. and Regier, D.A. Lifetime prevalence of specific disorders in three sites. *Archives of General Psychiatry* 1984; **41**:949-958.

13 Karno, M., Hough, R.L., Burnham, M.A. Escobar, J.I., Timbers, D.M., Santana, F. and Boyd, J.H. Lifetime prevalence of specific psychiatric disorders among Mexican Americans and non-Hispanic whites in Los Angeles. *Archives of General Psychiatry* 1987; **44**:695-701.

14 Burnham, M.A., Hough, R.L., Escobar, J.I., Karno, M., Timbers, D.M., Telles, C.A. and Locke, B.Z. Six month prevalence of specific psychiatric disorders among Mexican Americans and non-Hispanic whites in Los Angeles. *Archives of General Psychiatry* 1987; **44**:687-694.

15 Blazer, D., George, L.K., Landerman, R., Pennybacker, M., Melville, M.L., Woodbury, M., Manton, K.G., Jordan, K. and Locke, B. Psychiatric disorders: a rural/urban comparison. *Archives of General Psychiatry* 1985; **42**:651-656.

16 Canino, G.J., Bird, H.R., Shrout, P.E., Rubio-Stipec, M., Bravo, M., Martinez, R., Sesman, M. and Guevara, L.M. The prevalence of specific psychiatric disorders in Puerto Rico. *Archives of General Psychiatry* 1987; **44**:727-735.

17 Bland, R.C., Newman, S.C. and Orn, H. Epidemiology of psychiatric disorders in Edmonton. *Acta Psychiatrica Scandinavica,* 1988; **77**:Supplementum 338.

18 Hwu, H.-G., Yeh, E.-K. and Chang, L.-Y. Prevalence of psychiatric disorders in Taiwan defined by the Chinese Diagnostic Interview Schedule. *Acta Psychiatrica Scandinavica* 1989; **79:**136-147.

19 Regier, D.A., Boyd, J.H., Burke, J.D., Rae, D.S., Myers, J.K., Kramer, M., Robins, L.N., George, L.K., Karno, M. and Locke, B.Z. One month prevalence of mental disorders in the United States. *Archives of General Psychiatry* 1988; **45:**977-986.

20 Weissman, M.M., Leaf, P.J., Tischler, G.L., Blazer, D.G., Karno, M. Bruce, M.L. and Florio, M.P. Affective disorders in five United States communities. *Psychological Medicine* 1988; **18:**141-154.

21 Oakley-Browne, M.A., Joyce, P.R., Wells, J.E., Bushnell, J.A. and Hornblow, A.R. Christchurch Psychiatric Epidemiology Study, Part I: Six month and other period prevalences of specific psychiatric disorders. *Australian and New Zealand Journal of Psychiatry* 1989; **23:**327-340.

22 Wells, J.E., Bushnell, J.A., Hornblow, A.R., Joyce, P.R. and Oakley-Browne, M.A. Christchurch Psychiatric Epidemiology Study: Methodology and lifetime prevalence for specific psychiatric disorders. *Australian and New Zealand Journal of Psychiatry* 1989; **23:**315-326.

23 Bebbington, P.E. Population surveys of psychiatric disorder and the need for treatment. In press: *Social Psychiatry and Psychiatric Epidemiology* 1989.

24 Wing, J.K., Cooper, J.E. and Sartorius, N. *The Measurement and Classification of Psychiatric Symptoms.* Cambridge University Press: Cambridge 1974.

25 Bebbington, P., Hurry, J., Tennant, C., Sturt, E. and Wing, J.K. The epidemiology of mental disorders in Camberwell. *Psychological Medicine* 1981; **11:**561-80.

26 Sturt, E., Bibbington, P.E., Hurry, J. and Tennant, C. The Present State Examination used by interviewers from a Survey Agency: Report from the Camberwell Community Survey. *Psychological Medicine* 1981; **11:**185-192.

NEUROENDOCRINE RESPONSE TO SEROTONERGIC CHALLENGE IN OBSESSIVE COMPULSIVE DISORDER

Naomi Fineberg and Stuart A Montgomery
St Mary's Hospital Medical School, London

INTRODUCTION

Obsessive Compulsive Disorder (OCD) was once thought of as an uncommon psychiatric disorder, but is now recognised to be a rather more common psychiatric illness affecting some 2-3% of the population. It is a complex syndrome, characterised by a constellation of psychiatric symptoms, and is not simply a description of aberrant learnt behaviour. The illness tends to come on early in adulthood, affects males and females alike and, untreated, runs a long term chronic course with occasional exacerbations. Only a fraction of OCD sufferers come forward for medical help and therefore the illness is responsible for a great deal of morbidity in the population at large.

OCD is characterised by obsessional ruminations, which are recurrent, intrusive thoughts, and compulsive rituals, which are repetitive unwanted acts which the patients feels powerless to resist. These symptoms are distressing and socially disabling, and it is therefore not altogether surprising that patients often experience psychological and somatic symptoms of anxiety, and that the illness is often accompanied by symptoms of depression.

A serotonergic mechanism for OCD?

The strongest body of evidence favouring the serotonergic basis for OCD comes from the wealth of controlled treatment studies that have recently been performed in this area.[1] 5-HT uptake inhibitors have been found to be effective, whereas antidepressants without potent effects on the 5-HT system have not, which suggests that OCD is a serotonin specific illness.

The specificity of effect that was observed with 5-HT uptake inhibitors suggested that OCD would be a worthwhile target for the investigation of the underlying biological aspects of the illness, and the mechanism of therapeutic effect. OCD is a well defined syndrome and this has also encouraged the search for biological markers of serotonergic abnormalities. This paper considers the evidence from neuroendocrine probe work for the serotonergic basis of OCD.

The consistency of the clinical efficacy findings which generated the hypothesis that OCD is a serotonergic related illness, and which have provided the most compelling evidence of a serotonergic basis for the illness, is in contrast to the inconsistent results of studies which have sought biological markers of OCD or functional changes in neurotransmitter systems related to treatment. This may be due to the lack of apposite models and the use of inappropriate methodology. In animals, where direct measures of serotonergic function might be possible, there are no clear cut and accepted models of OCD; indirect measures in human subjects have to be used.

Neuroendocrine tests of 5-HT function in OCD

One of the more direct approaches to investigating serotonergic function has been the use of a neuroendocrine challenge test. A rise in plasma levels of pituitary hormones, eg prolactin, growth hormone and ACTH following administration of a serotonergic agent is taken as a measure of the integrity of the hypothalamic serotonergic system. Underactivity or overactivity of the central serotonin pathways would be reflected in a blunted or enhanced endocrine response. Serotonin function is assessed globally in one type of test that administers an agent which enhances serotonin release from terminals in a non-specific manner. A second type of test attempts to be more selective, by administering a specific 5-HT receptor agonist and assessing the integrity of the particular receptor to which the agonist binds.

For an ideal test the agent used in the challenge should be well tolerated, and have a clearly defined, selective serotonergic mechanism of action. It should reliably bring about an increase in hormone plasma levels following administration.[2] Unfortunately none of the methods available satisfy all these criteria.

A further problem with the neuroendocrine challenge model is the need for selectivity of effect. Other neurotransmitters than serotonin, eg dopamine, can cause the release of pituitary hormones, and to be sure that the test is a measure of serotonin function the compound used must be selective in its action. Some of the agents that have been used in neuroendocrine tests were thought to have selective serotonergic effects, but were shown later to have other actions as well. There should therefore be some hesitation in accepting too readily the claims for selectivity of some of the new compounds being developed, and thorough investigation is needed.

mCPP as a neuroendocrine challenge in OCD

One of the agents originally thought to be relatively serotonin-selective was the metabolite of trazodone, 1-m-chlorophenylpiperazine (mCPP). It now appears to act at 5-HT1A, 5-HT1B, 5-HT1C and 5-HT2 receptors, as well as being equipotent at alpha2 receptors and less potent at alpha1, dopamine and muscarinic receptors.[3] When it was first used as a neuroendocrine test these actions were not known and its effects on prolactin and cortisol, which could be blocked by metergoline, a 5-HT1 and 5-HT2 antagonist, seemed to recommend it as a suitable test.[4]

The two mCPP studies that attempted to detect an underlying serotonergic abnormality in OCD patients which would differentiate them from controls were both small, and the results inconsistent. One study[5] found a significantly lower increase in cortisol in patients with OCD compared with controls but no statistically significant difference in the mCPP-induced prolactin surge between the groups. The other study[6] found no difference in cortisol or growth hormone levels between patients and controls, but reported a significantly blunted prolactin surge in the OCD patients, although only in females.

It is difficult to know whether this lack of accord results from the unsuitability of mCPP as a serotonergic challenge agent or to differences in methodology.

L-Tryptophan Challenge in OCD

L-tryptophan administered intravenously is a more specific test of the serotonergic system than mCPP. A single small study comparing untreated OCD patients with controls has been performed[6] which demonstrates a significant enhancement of the prolactin response in the patient group. However, when each sex was examined independently a significant difference could no longer be found. While this finding provides some corroboration of the mCPP results, and suggests possible abnormalities in hypothalamic serotonin function in OCD, there is a clear risk in drawing conclusions from small studies which may not be able to take factors like sex differences in expected response into account.

Neuroendocrine tests in treated OCD

Another approach has been to investigate the serotonin status of OCD patients treated with 5-HT uptake inhibitors, the argument being that if treatment with a 5-HT uptake inhibitor produces serotonergic subsensitivity as an adaptive change, one might expect a decrease in the mCPP-induced prolactin response following treatment. This question was addressed in the study of Zohar et al[7] which repeated the mCPP challenge in obsessional patients following four months treatment with clomipramine. It was found that the sustained prolactin surge following mCPP challenge was not significantly different from the pre-treatment prolactin response.

Single-Dose Challenge in OCD Symptomatology

OCD symptoms, or changes in OCD symptoms appearing in response to a serotonergic challenge, have also been measured as a marker of serotonergic activity. These studies, which have usually investigated acute responses to single doses of various compounds, have a basic flaw: the inappropriate measurement of symptomatology. The sudden rapid changes measured in the acute single dose studies bear no relation to the clinical picture where response is measured over a reasonable period of time, and are most likely to represent immediate side effects of the drug administered.

Intravenous L-tryptophan was used a single dose challenge by Charney *et al*[6] and fenfluramine by Hollander *et al*[8] and in neither study were clinical changes seen in OCD symptomatology. This is not surprising since response in OCD, although faster than in depression, is not expected so rapidly. There is therefore some reservation about interpreting the increase in OCD symptoms following a single dose of mCPP and the decrease following placebo in OCD patients reported by Hollander *et al*,[8] particularly in view of the low placebo response which characterises OCD. The reported shortlived increases in anxiety and OCD symptoms in obsessional patients following a single oral dose of mCPP, which may be attenuated following successful treatment, are likewise difficult to interpret.[5,7]

mCPP is a drug with substantial side effects, eg nausea and anxiety, which makes it difficult, if not impossible, to preserve blindness in a single-dose comparison against placebo. The anxiety side effect is a particular problem with OCD patients who usually have anxiety symptoms as part of their obsessional illness. Any increase in anxiety may well appear, in a patient with OCD, as an increase in OCD symptoms. The problem of disentangling side effects from presumed receptor changes makes the single-dose study an inappropriate design, and studies of longer term treatment are needed.

5-HT antagonism and clinical response in OCD

Metergoline, a mixed 5-HT1 and 5-HT2 antagonist, has been investigated in untreated and treated OCD patients. Metergoline administration appeared to reverse the therapeutic response achieved by patients treated with clomipramine, and produced a rise in anxiety and OCD symptoms.[9] Metergoline is better tolerated than mCPP and this study gave repeated doses so that the criticisms of the acute single dose studies are less pertinent. The finding of a reversal of therapeutic effect cannot easily be attributed solely to the side effects of metergoline, as the behaviourial response was sustained, and increased with time.

This study appears to be a demonstration of the association between serotonergic activity and therapeutic effect in OCD. Because of the mixed effects of metergoline it is not possible to clarify whether the effect is mediated by 5-HT1 or 5-HT2 activity or a combination. Replication studies are, however, needed since an earlier study by Zohar *et al*[5] paradoxically found that single doses of metergoline appeared to improve obsessional symptoms in untreated patients.

More selective test compounds are needed

It is not yet known which are the more important 5-HT receptor subtypes in mediating clinical response in OCD, nor indeed which receptor subtypes are responsible for mediating hormone release. The involvement of 5-HT1A receptors is apparent but there is also good evidence that 5-HT1-like receptors and 5-HT2 receptors interact, and it is possible that the neuroendocrine response reflects this interaction.[10] The development of receptor-specific drugs should allow for a more sophisticated appraisal of 5-HT mechanisms in OCD. Unfortunately, there have been no controlled therapeutic trials, placebo or otherwise, in OCD for any of the currently available agents thought to be receptor-specific, and it is therefore not possible to make an informed guess about efficacy. The single open study with buspirone[11] is both small and subject to the bias inherent in open studies.

Different response mechanism in OCD and Depression

Neuroendocrine tests of 5-HT function have also been applied to the investigation of depression, and the results may have some bearing on the issue of the separation of OCD and depression. The earlier test yielded rather confusing results, which may have reflected a failure to adequately control for weight loss. For example, whereas blunted prolactin responses were measured following fenfluramine[12] and L-tryptophan challenge,[13] Meltzer et al[14] found the opposite effect, with an enhanced 5-OH tryptophan induced prolactin response in depressed individuals compared with healthy controls.

It was hard to reconcile these conflicting findings until it was demonstrated that weight loss independently enhanced L-tryptophan-mediated hormone responses in healthy dieters[15] and in depressed patients. Depressed patients who did not lose weight showed blunted hormone responses.[16]

More recent studies have supported this view, and indicate that, when weight loss is controlled for, patients with depression consistently show significantly blunted L-tryptophan-induced prolactin and growth hormone responses, suggesting a deficiency in hypothalamic 5-HT functions in depression.[17,18,19]

Treatment of depressed patients with fluvoxamine significantly enhanced the L-tryptophan induced endocrine responses, both after 1 week and 4 weeks of treatment. This enhancement of 5-HT function did not, however, correlate with clinical improvement, as antidepressant efficacy for fluvoxamine was not seen until the later stages. It appears that enhancement of 5-HT activity along is not responsible for the antidepressant effect of treatment, and it may be that adaptive changes at 5-HT receptors are required.[20] In OCD, the therapeutic response to 5-HT uptake inhibitors is rapid, with significant drug placebo differences as early as after only 1 or 2 weeks of treatment,[21,22,23] which may be too early for adaptive changes at 5-HT receptors to occur. This early response suggests that the mechanism of the antiobsessional effect differs from the antidepressant effect for 5-HT reuptake inhibitor drugs.

CONCLUSION

The studies of biological markers in OCD have generally not controlled for dose, and have made assumptions of an "all or none" receptor change being associated with efficacy. The interrelationship between receptors is likely to be more complex. The relationship between acute changes in symptoms on a single dose of a drug, which may in any case merely reflect side effects of the drug administered, and efficacy in chronic treatment has been inadequately investigated. The studies have been particularly hampered by the lack of drugs that are specific in their pharmacological action, for use as a challenge. Progress will depend on investigating in well conducted placebo controlled studies, whether some of the newer, more selective drugs used as probes are, indeed, selective for serotonin systems at particular doses, and in establishing separately, their efficacy. Only then will it be possible to infer whether changes in measures of particular 5-HT receptor subtypes are associated with response in OCD.

REFERENCES

1 Montogmery S A, Fineberg N, Montgomery D B. The efficacy of serotonergic drugs in OCD-power calculations compared with placebo. This issue.

2 Checkley S A. Neuroendocrine tests of monoamine function in man: A view of basic theory and its application to the study of depressive illness. *Psychol Med* 1980; **10**:35–53.

3 Hamik A and Peroutka S. 1-m-chlorophenylpiperazine (mCPP) interactions with neurotransmitter receptors in human brain. *Biol Psychiatry* 1989;**25**:569–575.

4 Mueller E A, Murphy P L, Sunderland T. Further studies of the putative serotonin against M-chlorophenyl piperazine: evidence for a serotonin receptor mediated mechanism of action in humans. *Psychopharmacology* 1986;**89**:388–391.

5 Zohar J, Mueller A, Insel T R, Zohar-Kadouch R C, Murphy D L. Serotonergic responsivity in obsession compulsive disorder: Comparison of patients and healthy controls. *Arch Gen Psychiatry* 1987;**44**:946–951.

6 Charney D S, Goodman W K, Price C H *et al*. Serotonin Function in Obsessive Compulsive Disorder. 1988;**45**:177–185.

7 Zohar J, Insel T, Zohar-Kadouch R, *et al*. Serotonergic responsivity in obsessive compulsive disorder. Effects of chronic clomipramine treatment. *Arch Gen Psychiatry* 1988;**45**:167–172.

8 Hollander E, Fay M, Cohen B *et al*. Serotonergic and noradrenergic sensitivity in obsessive compulsive disorder: behaviourial findings. *Am J Psychiatry* 1988;**145**:1015–1017.

9 C, Murphy D, Zohar J *et al*. Clomipramine in OCD: further evidence for a serotonergic mechanism of action. *Arch Gen Psych* 1989;**46**:23–28.

10 Charig E M, Anderson I M, Robinson J M *et al*. L-Tryptophan and prolactin release: evidence for interaction between 5-HT$_1$ and 5-HT$_2$ receptors. *Hum Psychopharmacol* 1986;**1**:93–97.

11 Jenike M A and Baer L. An open trial of Buspirone in obsessive compulsive disorder. *Am J Psychiatry* 1988;**145**:1285–1286.

12 Siever L J, Murphy D L, Slater S, De la Vega E, Lippen S. Plasma prolactin following fenfluramine in depressed patients compared to controls: an evaluation of central serotonergic responsivity in depression. *Life Sci* 1984;**34**:1029–1039.

13 Heninger G R, Charney D S, *et al*. Seronergic function in depression. *Arch Gen Psychiatry* 1984;**41**:398–402.

14 Meltzer H Y, Perline R, Tricou B J, Lowry M, Robertson A. Effect of hydroxy-tryptophan on serum cortisol levels in major affective disorders: Enhanced response in depression and mania. *Arch Gen Psychiatry* 1984;**41**:366–374.

15 Goodwin G M, Fairburn C G, Cowen P J. The effects of dieting and weight loss on neuroendocrine responses to L-typrophan clonidine and apomorphine in volunteers: important implications for neuroendocrine investigation in depression. *Arch Gen Psychiatry* 1987;**44**:952–5.

16 Cowen P J, Charig E. Neuroendocrine responses to tryprophan in major depression. *Arch Gen Psychiatry* 1987;**44**:958–966.

17 Koyoma T, Meltzer H Y. A biochemical and neuroendocrine study of the serotonergic system in depression. In: Hippius H *et al* (eds). New results in depression research. Springer-Verlag, Berlin. 1986:169–188.

18 Deakin J F W, Pennell I. 5-HT receptors sub types and depression. *Psychopharmacol* 1986;**89**:24.

19 Deakin J F W, Pennell I, *et al*. A neuroendocrine study of 5-HT function in depression: Evidence for biological mechanisms of endogenous and psychosocial causatien. 1990. (in press).

20 Price C H, Charney D S, Delgado *et al*. Effects of desipramine and fluvoxamine treatment on the prolactin response to tryptophan. *Arch Gen Psychiatry* 1989;**46**:625–631.

21 Montgomery S A. Clomipramine in obsessional neurosis: A placebo-controlled trial. *Pharm Med* 1980;**1**:(2), 189–192.

22 de Veaugh Geiss J, Landau P, Katz R. Treatment of obsessive compulsive disorder with clomipramine. *Psychiatr Ann* 1989;**19**:(2), 97–101.

23 Goodman W K, Price L H, Rasmussen S A *et al*. Efficacy of fluvoxamine in obsessive compulsive disorder. *Arch Gen Psychiatry* 1989;**46**:36–44.

COGNITIVE FACTORS IN OBSESSIVE-COMPULSIVE DISORDER

Paul M. Salkovikis

University of Oxford, Department of Psychiatry

INTRODUCTION

Psychological treatment for obsessional problems

Much of the interest in Obsessive compulsive disorder was generated by early work carried out in the area of psychological treatments, particularly that of Rachman, Marks, Hodgson and others. The reason for the early interest in this problem was because it was the most intractable of the neurotic disorders, with expectations being for a purely deteriorating course. Behavioural treatment has undoubtedly resulted in a radical improvement in prognosis, with a median success rate of 75%.[1,2] However, further developments in psychological treatment have been relatively slow, and a number of major problems remain to be resolved. Many of these problems apply not only to behaviour therapy but to all kinds of treatment, and require the use of specific research strategies if further progress is to be made. In this paper, the current status of psychological treatments is briefly reviewed, and the basis for the development of cognitive strategies is outlined. The implications of psychological analyses of obsessional problems for research in cognitive-behavioral and biological factors in OCD are considered, and specific therapeutic applications outlined.

Problems and developments in the treatment of obsessive compulsive disorder

Many patients refuse therapy altogether or drop out of treatment soon after it has started. Some patients do not improve with behaviour therapy, notably those with severe concurrent depression and obsessional "ruminators" (i.e. with no obvious compulsive behaviours). Finally, there is small but consistent relapse rate after the cessation of treatment. Of those patients suitable for and seeking treatment, *more than 50%* do not obtain a long term resolution of their problems.[3,4] Amongst the patients who do improve, outpatient treatment is sometimes lengthy and can be distressing to patients and therapists at times. Treatment may be incomplete, in that residual symptoms and handicap often persist after termination, although this is seldom measured properly.[5] It seems likely that the problems of treatment refusal and failure to respond to behavioural treatments apply equally to pharmacotherapy.

Thus, the way in which treatments are applied to obsessional problems needs to be extended to encompass those patients who do not benefit from currently available approaches. Even in fully compliant patients who are actively involved in treatment, it would undoubtedly be helpful to find ways of conducting treatment more efficiently and effectively. There has only been one major recent development in this respect. In terms of cost-effectiveness, it has now been clearly demonstrated that the widely adopted clinical practice of conducting exposure with response prevention (ERP) on an outpatient rather than inpatient basis is indeed justified in terms of effectiveness of treatment.[6] Marks demonstrated the crucial role of self-exposure homework; it is possible that, for some obsessional patients, self-exposure homework will be *more* effective than therapist aided exposure. The results of studies of the efficacy of self-directed exposure were crucially important because almost all of the key studies of ERP had previously been conducted on an impatient basis. However, this helps with cost rather than effectiveness, and clinical experience suggests that problems with compliance and treatment refusal are not solved by self-exposure homework. In order to understand the nature of the problems, it is helpful to reconsider the theoretical basis of existing psychological treatment.

The behavioural theory of obsessional problems

Behavioural accounts of obsessive-compulsive disorder propose that ritualistic behaviour is crucial to the maintenance of obsessions.[2] Ritualistic behaviour prevents the patients from getting used to upsetting thoughts ("habituating") by substantially shortening the period during which exposure to the thought occurs.[7] Stated formally, obsessions are said to have their origins in normal thinking, specifically as normal intrusive thoughts. Such thoughts become associated with anxiety as a result of learning; this learning can arise from direct experience or, as is more likely in this instance, through indirect learning from others (e.g. modelling or imitative learning, through specific teaching and so on). Behavioural theory can be specified in terms of its key points; thus:
(i) obsessions are thoughts with which anxiety has become associated and has subsequently failed to extinguish; (ii) patients develop responses (obsessional rituals or compulsions) which either avoid or terminate exposure to the stimuli; the compulsive behaviours persist because they are rewarded ("negatively reinforced") by the omission or reduction of anxiety or discomfort that they have come to expect will follow the occurrence of obsessional thinking; (iii) When patients avoid things which might trigger upsetting thoughts and use compulsive behaviours to "switch off" these thoughts, they not only stop themselves from feeling uncomfortable but also prevent themselves from experiencing the natural reduction in anxiety which occur if they did not avoid or use compulsive rituals.
This formulation helps to understand why obsessional behaviour, whilst feeling as if it is helpful and necessary from the patient's perspective, persists and has a major negative impact as a result of the way in which it prevents habituation of distress.

The role of overt compulsive behaviour as a key variable in the maintenance of obsessions has been demonstrated by experimental work by Rachman and his colleagues.[8,9,10] These experiments highlighted the importance of prolonged exposure with response prevention as a key mechanism of change.

Some problems: not so serious and serious

An important implication of the behavioural hypothesis is that obsessional thoughts *not* accompanied by compulsive behaviour should be extremely easy to treat or should not even exist, because the primary maintaining factor (compulsive behaviour) is not present. This conclusion is *not* borne out by the treatment outcome data for obsessional ruminations (obsessional thoughts without overt compulsive behaviours). Ruminations are more difficult to treat than obsessive-compulsive disorder.[11] Rachman[4] summarised the position as "The main obstacle to the successful treatment of obsessions is the absence of effective techniques". Thus, ruminations are particularly distressing and highly resistant to existing treatment, although theoretically they should spontaneously remit or require only minimal treatment.

This apparently serious challenge to the basis of the behavioural theory can be dealt with by a simple modification. The term "rumination" as applied to the mental activity of patients without overt compulsive behaviours can be divided into intrusive thoughts and *neutralising thoughts,* which are the mental equivalent of compulsive behaviour.[11] The equivalence is functional, in that neutralising thoughts can be regarded as fulfilling the same function as overt compulsive behaviour (i.e. they terminate exposure to obsessional thoughts and therefore prevent habituation taking place). The defining characteristic of covert neutralising is not the content (which may in some instances be identical to that of the obsessional thoughts which trigger neutralising), but instead is to be found in the fact that neutralising responses are intentional acts. The voluntary nature of neutralising contrasts with the intrusive, unwanted and involuntary nature of obsessional intrusions. Treatment therefore requires response prevention of neutralising, and the problem is reduced to terms understandable from existing behavioural perspectives, although there are clearly some special difficulties involved in response prevention of an "invisible" ritual (see[12] for a fuller account of treatment procedures).

The inclusion of this cognitive component raises the question of the role of cognitive factors in obsessional problems. The potential usefulness of the cognitive approach to a wide range of problems such as depression, panic, generalised anxiety, social anxiety and so on is now well cognised, and it could reasonably be hoped that similar advances might be possible for obsessional disorders.

The cognitive view may help to account for a number of observations are not readily explained by the behavioural approach and which therefore present serious problems for the hypothesis. These include the following findings:

(1) Some patients show increases in anxiety when they ritualise.[13,2]
(2) Discomfort experienced when an obsession is provoked can be decreased by the presence of the therapist in patients with checking rituals, but not in patients with contamination and washing rituals.[8,9,10]
(3) The prevalence of reassurance seeking as a ritual in washers, checkers and ruminators[1,14] cannot be accounted for by the behavioural mode.
(4) The obvious relationship between depressed mood and obsessional problems has yet to be accounted for in a satisfactory fashion.[13,2] Such observations suggest that at the very least, the behavioural hypothesis is not sufficiently detailed.

Most problematic of all is the lack of specificity of the behavioural hypothesis, particularly the extent to which it fails to distinguish between obsessions, normal intrusive phenomena and phobias. The aetiological view of obsessions, like that of phobias, is based on the idea of the acquisition of a conditioned fear response, interacting with developmental and biological factors.[15] Compared with phobias (for which the conditioning approach was first evoked), it transpires that obsessional thoughts are a more widespread phenomenon amongst the normal population than was originally supposed, with around 90% of normal subjects reporting their occurrence.[16,17] There is apparently nothing in the immediate characteristics of such normal intrusions to distinguish between these and obsessional thoughts in a clinical population. However, there is also little to distinguish between the behavioural account of obsessions and that of phobias.[18,19] In both instances, a key role is played by avoidance and escape behaviours which are hypothesised to prevent the extinction of conditioned fear. Sensitivity to criticism is one of the few variables which has been shown to differentiate obsessionals and phobics.[2] The possible importance of cognitive factors is highlighted by Marks[7], who pointed out that: "obsessives develop a more elaborate set of beliefs around their rituals than phobics develop around their fears. Cognitions seem to play a larger role in obsessives than in phobics. Minor changes in obsessives' perception of a situation can therefore produce a marked change in their behaviour." [p40].

The foundations of the cognitive approach to obsessions

Behaviour therapists have always taken account of cognitive factors to some extent. In particular, the work of Lang[20] and its adoption by Rachman & Hodgson[21] suggested that there should be a multi-faceted conceptualisation of anxiety. In particular, the division into behavioural, physiological and cognitive components of anxious responding was proposed. It was suggested that any patient would show a pattern of such responses, which may not be in perfect synchrony, especially during the course of treatment. For example, the patient may show reduced anxiety in the behavioural system (e.g. by approaching the feared stimulus) but show an increase in subjective anxiety and anxious thoughts. The adoption of three systems (rather than 30 systems or even 300) is a matter of simplicity rather than theoretically crucial; the important factor identified was that anxiety is not a "lump", and needs to be viewed as a complex set of imperfectly inter-related responses. Thus, a full understanding of obsessional problems requires consideration of a range of interacting factors rather than an assessment of symptoms of a unitary disorder.

A further and more recent development of this view is that some of the inter-relationships between response systems are, in fact, functional. That is, the response systems do not merely passively interact, but can be causally linked. The cognitive theory develops the idea of functional inter-relationships whilst at the same time taking account of the extensive and important work on behavioural and pharmacological approaches to the understanding and treatment of obsessional problems. Thus, the importance of developing a *cognitive*-behavioural hypothesis is twofold. Firstly, a more comprehensive understanding of the mechanisms involved in the origin and maintenance of obsessional problems may allow a more detailed analysis of the mode of action of other treatment modalities such as pharmacotherapy. Secondly, a cognitive-behavioural hypothesis might be expected to lead to the direct development of novel treatment strategies to make therapy faster, easier, more efficient and more enduring.[22,23]

Figure 1

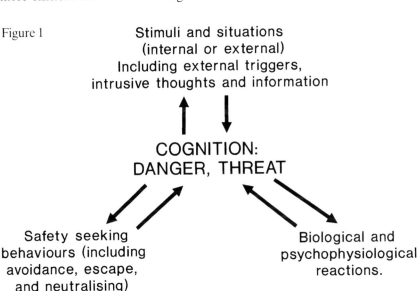

Stimuli and situations
(internal or external)
Including external triggers,
intrusive thoughts and information

COGNITION:
DANGER, THREAT

Safety seeking
behaviours (including
avoidance, escape,
and neutralising)

Biological and
psychophysiological
reactions.

The general cognitive model of anxiety is shown in Figure 1.[24] As must inevitably be the case for any theory of anxiety (psychological or biological) in which specific stimuli are considered to be relevant, the person's perception and interpretation (appraisal) of their internal and external environment is central. In order to be responsive to stimuli, information must be input and made sense of. Furthermore, this connection is two way, in the sense that the person's reaction to their environment will, in turn, provoke responses which can alter the way they perceive it. For example, when an anxiety provoking stimulus is detected the person may focus their attention on the more threatening aspects of it. The appraisal has effects on behaviour and on biological/psychophysiological reactions; as is well known, both types of reactions can, in turn, have an effect on the perception of threat. Thus, a central component of anxiety problems is the thinking pattern involved in the input of information; this can set up a complex series of interactions which will be affected by a range of predispositions (cognitive, biological and behavioural) with obsessional disorders resulting in some instances.

Components of a cognitive-behavioural analysis

Thus, the cognitive analysis suggests that a central feature is the way in which the thoughts or obsessional stimuli are appraised (i.e. judged, interpreted, appraised and analysed). This appraisal determines the emotional response; a *generally* negative appraisal is not the cognitive component of obsessional disorders, and simply tends to result in anxiety or depression. The specific obsessional appraisal concerns responsibility. If one regards a thought as reflecting immediate responsibility for action, this produces both discomfort and a tendency to take remedial action in the form of neutralising or ritualising behaviour.

Origins of intrusive thoughts

Thus, some individuals are vulnerable to interpreting intrusive thoughts as indicating that they may be in a position to prevent harm to themselves or to other people (i.e. overperceive their responsibility). It is likely that such individuals have been socialised into being particularly sensitive *vis a vis* the degree of responsibility they have when they experience intrusive thoughts. This sensitivity is best described as exaggerated assumptions about the extent to which actual harm can result from thoughts themselves (e.g. "Having a thought about an action can lead you to carry out that action"), about the extent of responsibility for preventing harm (e.g. "Once you have thought about it, failing to prevent or failing to try to prevent harm is the same as having caused the harm"), or about the importance of ensuring that one is completely free of responsibility for harm to oneself or others (e.g. "If you have any doubt at all that you may have caused harm, then you *must* act to ensure that you are clear of blame"). A good summary of such beliefs can be found in what is described as a "thinking error", namely the assumption that having some *influence* over potential harm to oneself or others is identical to *being responsible for it*.

These and similar beliefs are particularly likely to begin to interact with intrusive thoughts after the occurrence of a critical incident which activates the assumptions. Critical incidents will generally (but not invariably) involve an element of increased responsibility or increases in perceived responsibility (for example, having a baby, the occurrence of an electrical fire in the patient's house, seeing news items about potentially harmful circumstances in everyday

31

Figure 2

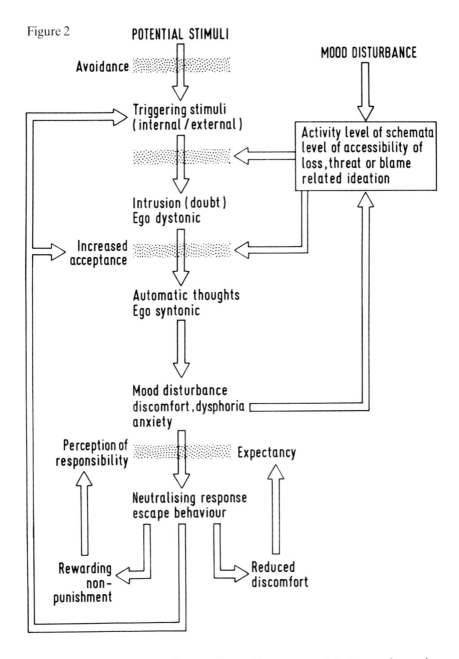

life). Such occurrences can have a direct effect on mood, but may also make individuals more likely to react to intrusive thoughts by *negative automatic thoughts* that their actions (or inaction) may make them responsible for harm to themselves or others. By definition, these automatic thoughts are plausible and believable, so that the individual is likely to respond with anxiety and *by taking precautions or corrective measures* to reduce or eliminate responsibility.

Maintenance of obsessional thoughts

It is the occurrence of negative automatic thoughts, avoidant behaviour and neutralising behaviour which is hypothesised to be involved in the maintenance of obsessions and to distinguish them from normal intrusive thoughts. In clinical obsessions, negative automatic thoughts of responsibility and neutralising behaviour (over or covert) will be more extensive than in non-clinical cases. (The implications of this part of the hypothesis are described in greater detail by Salkovskis[25,26] and Salkovskis & Warwick.[27] Figure 2 shows the way in which it is suggested that neutralising interacts with appraisal in obsessional disorder.

The mood and current concerns of the individual can increase both the frequency of occurrence of intrusive thoughts and the likelihood that such intrusions will be interpreted in a particularly negative way. Only when intrusive thoughts are interpreted negatively and result in negative automatic thoughts concerning blame will anxiety *and* neutralising result. That is, the intrusive thought has to be interpreted as having important implications for the behaviour of the patient for neutralising to result; if free of such implications, discomfort or distress may result, but not neutralising. Without neutralising, the mechanism will be very similar to those outlined by Teasdale[28] in the maintenance of depressed mood, accounting for the strength of the depression/obsessions association. Neutralising maintains the obsessional pattern in several ways; it prevents the patient from disconfirming their fears of harm, it increases the acceptance of worries about responsibility, and makes the obsessional thought the subject of further detailed cognitive processing (and hence increases both the current pre-occupation and the future salience of the thought; see below). Neutralising itself can also be maintained by anxiety reduction where this takes place, although it seems likely that the more potent maintaining factor is the perceived reduction in the *risk of being responsible for harm*. Thus, obsessive-compulsive disorder can be seen as being on a continuum with normal intrusive thoughts, with the degree of neutralising (and the intensity of the corresponding automatic thoughts concerning responsibility) determining the position along the continuum rather than the intensity, frequency or uncontrollability of the intrusive thoughts.

Obsessional disorders are thus the outcome of the interplay of a range of inter-related factors. Better understanding of these complex interactions will benefit treatments of any kind. It seems likely that different treatments have their beneficial effects by acting on the components of obsessions and the interactions between them; however, those working with any particular modality cannot afford to ignore the way in which other systems may impinge. This is so whether the specific schema identified is cognitive, neurochemical, behavioural or biological; it is no longer sensible to regard any component of the complex of factors in obsessional problems in isolation.

Obsessional problems can be analysed in terms of the interaction between a potentially vulnerable organism and a complex environment. A range of new and more meaningful questions are available to researchers. For example: at what level is fluvoxamine having an effect? The fact that it has a beneficial effect means that it must be having some impact on subjective anxiety; does it have specific effects on ritualising, on thought rituals, on the perception of the environment, on the intrusiveness of upsetting thoughts, on the frequency of intrusive thoughts, on how upsetting they are?

It is also evident that the complexity of our analysis of such factors may need to increase. At the behavioural level, for example, it is important to consider ritualistic behaviour, mental neutralising and deliberate attempts at thought suppression.[29] Each has been shown to be important in the perpetuation of intrusive thoughts. The paradoxical effects of though suppression, in which trying *not* to think a particular thought makes it more likely that one will, is especially interesting in consideration of the frequency of upsetting thoughts. Obsessional patients try very hard to suppress distressing thoughts; is this tendency affected by different treatments? It seems likely that pharmacological treatments do not target specific fears, but rather have their effect by changing generalised behavioural or cognitive tendencies. It seems vital to know more about such effects. If such relationships can be clarified, it should indicate the best ways to combine treatments in order to minimise or prevent relapse at the end of treatment, or even to optimise the impact of the treatment themselves. How do the systems involved in obsessional disorders interact and how do treatments affect such interactions? More sophisticated research into the mechanisms by which obsessional problems are maintained are urgently required.

CONCLUSION

Summary and therapeutic implications

The development of psychological approaches to the treatment of obsessions and compulsions has stimulated much important research and generated the conditions for the development of a range of new treatments. Psychological approaches have themselves continued to develop; cognitive therapy is a particularly promising possible adjunct to existing behavioural treatments. Cognitive treatment is based on a specific account of the origins and maintenance of obsessions: (i) that obsessional thoughts are the same type of cognition as intrusive thoughts in normal subjects; (ii) that distress arises not from the intrusive thought itself but from the way in which it is interpreted; (iii) that the persistence of intrusive thoughts and their distressing interpretation result from the occurrence of *neutralising activity* (mental or actual rituals); (iv) that neutralising occurs when the occurrence of the intrusive thought is interpreted as meaning that the patient is responsible for taking preventative action against harm to self or others.

This formulation suggests several points at which treatment might be effective; (i) in helping the patient find ways of blocking all neutralising activity

34

(overt *and* covert); (ii) in changing the way in which thoughts are interpreted, particularly by reducing perception of responsibility for harm.

Applications of cognitive therapy could include (a) Facilitating assessment (b) An alternative to exposure; (c) Ensuring compliance with exposure; (d) Facilitating re-appraisal during exposure; (e) Generalising treatment; (f) Treating associated mood disturbance; (g) Treating overvalued ideation.

The focus of cognitive-behavioural treatment is thus on helping the patient to identify and modify overt or covert neutralising responses, assumptions concerning responsibility and modification of the way in which the occurrence of intrusive thoughts is interpreted by the patient.

Psychological treatments have several characteristics which make them highly appropriate for use in the treatment of obsessions. Probably because treatment aims to bring about permanent changes in factors which maintain the patients' problems, behavioural and cognitive-behavioural treatments have generally been shown to have better long-term outcome on the cessation of treatment as compared with medication.[30] Combinations are, of course, well worth investigating for this reason. An important feature of the well defined treatments which characterise behavioural and cognitive behavioural therapy is the way in which they can be adapted and improved, by both adding new components and shortening to make them more efficient (see, for example, discussion of self exposure above). It seems likely that the already effective treatments used for obsessional problems will be refined further over the next decade, and adapted for use with a wider patient population. Recent developments improving the efficiency of treatment mean that the cost of psychological therapies is low when considered in the context of the timescale involved, which tends to be between eight and fifteen sessions of therapy. Perhaps most significantly of all, work on the normal basis of obsessional problems opens exciting new possibilities for prevention, which is, of course, likely to be least costly option of all.

ACKNOWLEDGEMENTS

The author is grateful to the Medical Research Council of the United Kingdom for their support.

REFERENCES

1 Marks, I.M. *Fears, phobias and rituals.* Oxford University Press, New York. 1987
2 Rachman, S.J., & Hodgson, R. *Obsessions and compulsions.* Englewood Cliffs, NJ: Prentice Hall. 1980.
3 Foa, E.B., Steketee, G., Grayson, J.B., & Doppelt, H.G. Treatment of obsessive-compulsives: when do we fail? In: E.B. Foa & P.M.G. Emmelkamp eds. *Failures in behaviour therapy.* New York: Wiley. 1983.
4 Rachman, S.J. Obstacles to the successful treatment of obsessions. In: E.B. Foa & P.M.G. Emmelkamp eds. *Failures in behaviour therapy.* New York: Wiley. 1983.

5 Jacobsen, N.S., Follettew, W.C., & Revenstorf, D. Psychotherapy outcome research: methods for reporting variability and evaluating clinical significance. *Behav Ther* 1984;**11**:336–352.

6 Marks, I.M., Lelliott, P., Basoglu, M., Noshirvani, H. Clomipramine, self exposure and therapist aided exposure in obsessive-compulsive ritualisers. *Br J Psychiatry et al* 1988;**152**:522–534.

7 Marks I.M. *Cure and care of neurosis*. New York: Wiley. 1981.

8 Rachman, S.J., de Silva, P., & Roper, G. The spontaneous decay of compulsive urges. *Behav Res Ther* 1976;**14**:445–453.

9 Roper, G., Rachman, S.J., & Hodgson, R. An experiment on obsessional checking. *Behav Res Ther* 1973;**11**:271–277.

10 Roper, G., & Rachman, S.J. Obsessional-compulsive checking: replication and development. *Behav Res Ther* 1975;**13**:25–32.

11 Salkovskis, P.M. and Westbrook, D. Behaviour therapy and obsessional ruminations: can failure be turned into success? *Behav Res Ther* 1989;**27**:149–160.

12 Salkovskis, P.M., and Kirk, J. Obsessional problems. In: K. Hawton, P.M. Salkovskis, J. Kirk and D.M. Clark eds. *Cognitive behaviour therapy for psychiatric problems: a practical guide*. Oxford: Oxford University Press. 1989.

13 Beech, H.R., & Liddel, A. Decision making, mood states and ritualistic behaviour among obsessional patients. In: H.R. Beech ed. *Obsessional States*. London: Methuen. 1974.

14 Warwick, H.M.C. & Salkovskis, P.M. Reassurance. *Br Med J* 1985;**290**:1028.

15 McNally, R.J. Preparedness and phobias: a review. *Psychol Bull* 1987;**101**:283-303.

16 Rachman, S.J. & de Silva, P. Abnormal and normal obsessions. *Behav Res Ther* 1978;**16**:233–238.

17 Salkovskis, P.M. & Harrison, J. Abnormal and normal obsessions – a replication. *Behav Res Ther* 1984;**22**:549–552.

18 Rachman, S.J. The passing of the two stage theory of fear and avoidance. *Behav Res Ther* 1976b;**14**:125–131.

19 Rachman, S.J. The conditioning theory of fear acquisition: a critical examination. *Behav Res Ther* 1977;**15**:375–387.

20 Lang, P.J. Stimulus control, dresponse control and the desensitisation of fear. In: *Learning approaches to therapeutic behaviour*. D.J. Levis ed. Chicago: Aldine Press. 1970.

21 Rachman, S.J., and Hodgson, R. Synchrony and desynchrony in fear and avoidance *Behav Res Ther* 1974;**12**:311–318.

22 Salkovskis, IP.M. & Westbrook, D. Obsessive-compulsive disorder: clinical strategies for improving behavioural treatmernts. In: H.R. Dent ed. *Clinical Psychology: research and development*. London: Croom Helm. 1987.

23 Salkovskis, P.M. Obsessive and intrusive thoughts: clinical and non-clinical aspects. In: eds. P.M.G. Emmelkamp, W.T.A.M. Everaerd, and M.J.M. van Son, *Fresh perspectives on anxiety disorders*. Amsterdam: Swets and Zeitlinger. 1989.

24 Beck, A.T., Emergy, G., and Greenberg, R. *Anxiety disorders and phobias: a cognitive perspective* Basic Books: New York. 1985.

25 Salkovskis, P.M. Obsessional-compulsive problems: a cognitive-behavioural analysis. *Behav Res Ther* 19854;**23**:571–583.

26 Salkovskis, P.M. Cognitive-behavioural factors and the persistence of intrusive thoughts in obsessional problems. *Behav Res Ther* 1989a;**27**:677–682.

27 Salkovskis, P.M., & Warwick, H.M.C. Cognitive therapy of obsessive-compulsive disorder. In: C. Perris, I.M. Blackburn & H. Perris eds. *The Theory and Practice of Cognitive Therapy*. 1988.

28 Teasdale, J.D. Negative thinking in depression: Cause, effect or reciprocal relationship? *Adv Behav Res Ther* 1983;**5**:3–25.

29 Salkovskis, P.M. Obsessions and compulsions. In: J. Scott, J.M.G. Williams & A.T. Beck eds. *Cognitive therapy: a clinical casebook*. Croom Helm: London. 1989b.

30 Clark, D.M. Cognitive treatments for depression and anxiety: is it better than drugs in the long term? In: K. Hawton and P. Cowan eds. *Dilemmas in Psychiatry*. Oxford University Press: Oxford. 1990.

A CONTROLLED STUDY OF FLUVOXAMINE AND EXPOSURE IN OBSESSIVE-COMPULSIVE DISORDER

Jean Cottraux

Neurological Hospital, Lyon, France

INTRODUCTION

Many authors have recommended serotonergic antidepressants for obsessive-compulsive disorder. However, their use raises some problems. Drug effects do not last beyond a few months, relapses are common after drug withdrawal[1] and side-effects can be a problem.[2] Some arguments exist in favour of a specific effect of serotonergic antidepressants in obsessive compulsive disorder[3], but non-serotonergic drugs have been little studied.

The relationship between drug effect and depression is complex.[4] Decrease in rituals with clomipramine does not correlate with baseline depression in children[5], or in non-depressed adults[6], but does in depressed adults.[7] When antiexposure instructions were given together with clomipramine the drug effect disappeared.[6] Exposure and response prevention is helpful, and is sufficient treatment for most non-depressed obsessive-compulsive subjects, with the improvement continuing up to 2-6 year follow up.[8,4] Clinicians need to take into account effectiveness, duration and cost of any given treatment, and of possible alternatives.

To address such issues we designed a controlled study of fluvoxamine, a potent and selective serotonin re-uptake inhibitor[9] versus placebo; both groups had exposure. In the third group we tried to test fluvoxamine and antiexposure. We report here outcome to week 48. No drug was taken in the follow up period after week 24. The dexamethasone suppression test data have been reported in a separate paper.[10] Side effects, predictors, and MMPI data will be reported in forthcoming papers.

METHODS

Study design

Three groups of 20 out-patients each were compared in a parallel randomised design:

Group I (F):   Fluvoxamine and Antiexposure Therapy.
Group II (Fe):   Fluvoxamine and Exposure Therapy.
Group III (Pe): Placebo and Exposure Therapy.

Fe and Pe groups were double-blind, while the F group was single-blind.

Full double-blindness would require a fourth group: placebo with antiexposure, which is not acceptable ethically. Comparison of F and Fe groups tested the effectiveness of exposure since fluvoxamine intake was comparable in both. Similarly, comparison of Fe and Pe groups tested the effectiveness of fluvoxamine since exposure level was comparable in both groups.

Sample

All patients had to meet DSM-III[11] criteria for obsessive-compulsive disorder initially. A 15 day wash-out period, during which only low dose bromazepam was taken, preceded the biological and behavioural assessments. A secondary diagnosis of major depression was acceptable, if it had been preceded by obsessive compulsive disorder. Typically patients said that depression was triggered by obsessive thoughts and compulsive rituals which led to a sense of helplessness and to work and marital maladjustment. Patients with Gilles de la Tourette syndrome, organic mental disorders and schizophrenia were excluded from the trial. MAOIs, barbiturates, clormethiazole, phenothiazines, butyrophenones, and neuroleptics were prohibited during the trial. Benzodiazepines were also prohibited, with the exception of intermittent bromazepam at up to 6 mg/day. Patients who required additional treatment to that allowed for in the group to which they had been randomly assigned were excluded, and counted as a failure for that group. All the patients signed an informed consent form before entering the study.

All but two patients had received pharmacotherapeutic agents in the years preceding the trial (anxiolytics, lithium, neuroleptics, hypnotics, or antidepressants alone or in combination). Fifty-one had experienced failure of antidepressant treatment. Ten had received ECT. Twelve patients were failures of the psychodynamic treatments of psychoanalysis and three had received behaviour therapy without success. Two patients presented with pure obsessions, while 58 had both obsessions and compulsions.

Of the 44 treatment completers 16 were men and 28 women. Mean age was 36 and mean duration of obsessive compulsive disorder was 13 years, so the group was very chronic.

Treatments

Medication was prescribed by a psychiatrist, while psychological treatment was administered by a different therapist. Patients took fluvoxamine at a dose of up to 300 mg, nocte, for 24 weeks and were seen by the psychiatrist 9 times after the initial session: at weeks 1, 2, 3, 4, 8, 12, 16, 20, 24. Medication was tapered off from weeks 24 to 28.

Psychological treatment

Exposure was divided into two periods in F and Fe groups: exposure homework and flooding in fantasy for the first 8 weeks, followed by guided exposure and response prevention for a further 16 weeks. The therapy format was flexible. Couple therapy, cognitive restructuring, flooding in fantasy, and assertive training were added as needed. By week 24 patients had had up to 25 sessions guided by four therapists. The therapists did not discuss the patients with the assessor and the prescribing psychiatrist.

For antiexposure patients were asked by the prescribing psychiatrist to avoid any kind of exposure to feared situations, to relax at a fixed period daily, and to let the rituals and/or obsessive thoughts just happen. They were given a short explanatory manual. Antiexposure was presented as a "mild form of behaviour therapy using relaxation instead of confrontation to feared situations". Antiexposure homework was checked at week 1, 2, 3, 4, 8, 12, 16, 20 and 24.

Measures

There were both self-ratings (S) and ratings by an assessor (A) who was blind to the treatment group and did not take part in treatment. Blindness was not tested by asking the assessor at the end to guess what treatment the patient had had. All ratings were made at week 0, 24 and 48 unless otherwise stated.

Rituals

(1) and (2). Four Target Rituals (S, A) were rated for time and discomfort (each on a 0-8 scale, yielding total score ranges of 0-32 for time and for discomfort).

(3) Total duration of rituals per day (S, A), (range 0-8). A reduction of more than 30% in this measure became:

(4) The criterion of ritual improvement (S), and a general criterion of improvement.[12] The total duration of rituals per day (S) reflected the interference of the rituals with patient's everyday life and, thus, was taken as the global criterion of treatment effectiveness. A reduction of more than 30% meant improvement.

Additional self-ratings on these 4 measures of rituals were made at week 8.

(5) Behavioural Avoidance Test (BAT) (S).[13] This involved four homework assignments given by the assessor to test avoidance (range 0-4) and discomfort (range 0-32) when confronting external or internal feared situations.

(6) Compulsion checklist, (S) (14; 13), score range 0-111.

Depression

(1) Beck Depression Inventory 13 items[15], (S), (range 0-39).
(2) Hamilton Rating Scale for Depression 17-items, (A), (range 0-52).
(3) Retardation Scale[16], (A), (range 0-56).
(4) MADRS[17], (A), (range 0-60).

Negative expectations were rated at week 0 on a 0 to 8 scale (S), both for exposure and fluvoxamine treatments.

Life events

An unvalidated French version of Andrews life events scale (S), (range 0-90) was filled-in at week 0 only.

Reliability

The Pearson product-moment correlation (df = 58) was computed to check the reliability of the self versus assessor-evaluated four target rituals forms. At week 0 the correlation coefficient r was 0.89 for total duration of rituals per day, 0.74 for target rituals discomfort, and 0.85 for target rituals time. At week 24 self versus assessor reliability was even higher: ritual total duration per day r = 0.91, target ritual discomfort r = 0.95 and time r = 0.95.

Compliance

Compliance with psychological treatment was evaluated:
(a) By counting the number of attended sessions, expressed as a percentage.
(b) By counting the number of completed homework tasks recorded by the patient in the homework diary from week 0-24, expressed as a percentage.

Compliance with drug treatment was evaluated by counting the number of pills taken from week 0-24, expressed as a percentage. In addition, a platelet serotonin assay (18) at week 0 and 24 was used as a global measure of compliance with the drug regimen.

Statistics

Statistical tests for non-parametric data were used because distributions of the scores were skewed. Within-group comparisons were made with Wilcoxon matched paired signed ranks test (two tailed). Between group comparisons used Chi-square for discontinuous variables with Yates correction, and Fisher exact probability test when cell frequencies were low. Continuous variables were compared among the three groups with Kruskal Wallis one-way ANOVA (two tailed). When differences were significant multiple paired between-group comparisons used Mann-Whitney U-tests (two tailed). Correlations between rating scales were calculated with Pearson product-moment correlation coefficient and Spearman rank correlation coefficient. Hotelling's T^2 was used

to make a global between group comparison of the variables.
Separate analyses were made for:
(1) Fifty patients having data for weeks 0-8.
(2) Forty-four patients (completers) having data for weeks 0-24.
(3) Thirty-seven patients having data for weeks 24-48.

RESULTS

Refusers and dropouts

Of 65 patients offered treatment 60 entered the trial, 50 reached week 8, 44 completed treatment to week 24, and 37 reached follow up to week 48. Ten patients dropped out between week 0 and week 8 (5 in the F group, 3 in the Fe group, and 2 in the Pe group: CHi^2 (df 2) – 1.68, p = 0.43).

Sixteen subjects (26%) did not complete the treatment (7 in the F group, 4 in the Fe group and 5 in the Pe group: CHi^2 (df 2) = 1.193, not statistically significant (NS). Dropouts at week 24 did not differ from completers for age, sex, expectations, life events, measures of depression, and obsessive compulsive disorder (data available upon request).

Reasons for dropping out at week 24 were as follows:

F group: four patients dropped out because they were not satisfied by their randomisation to antiexposure, one had an acute psychotic episode, and two due to drug side effects.

Fe group: One was withdrawn from the study because of suicidal thoughts, two due to drug side effects and one went abroad.

Pe group: three patients were withdrawn from the study becuase of suicidal thoughts, one due to treatment non-compliance and one because of placebo side effects.

Compliance

Compliance was studied in the 44 completers. Attendance to sessions was good: F = 99%, Fe = 99% and Pe = 98%: Kruskal-Wallis H = 1.33, df 2, p = 0.51. Complete record of the pills taken was available in 35 patients. Compliance was high and no difference was found between the three groups (F : 97%, Fe : 91% and Pe : 97%: Druskal-Wallis H = 0.511, df 2, p = 0.77). Thus, the drug versus placebo comparison appears valid. Moreover there was a significant decrease of platelet serotonin in both F and Fe groups compared with the Pe groups, while no statistical difference was found between F and Fe groups. No between group difference was found at week 0. This reflects a global compliance as shown by the following platelet serotonin values, mean ($\pm$ SD) : week 0 : F = 3.04 (1.3), Fe = 3.31 (1.65), Pe = 2.96 (1.01); week 24 : F = 0.42 (0.55), Fe = 1.34 (1.82), Pe = 3.86 (1.42).

Discontinuous use of bromazepam (2 to 6 mg) was allowed in 10 patients in the F group, 10 in the Fe group, and 6 in the Pe group. No between group difference appeared: Chi^2 (df 2) = 4.04, p = 0.132.

Compliance with exposure homework was good: 70% in the Fe group, and 78% in the Pe group. In contract compliance with antiexposure home-works in the F group was 25% : Kruskal-Wallis H (df 2) = 20.13, p < 0.001, with a significant exposure versus antiexposure effect in paired multiple comparisons : p = 0.0002. It was very hard to convince antiexposure patients to do relevant homework; most did none, having heard broadcasts about, read about or been told about exposure by their doctors and others. Four patients in the F group who dropped out said they did so because they were dissatisfied with the treatment. They had probably guessed that they had been assigned to a control group. Thus the comparison between exposure and antiexposure which it had been intended to make is probably invalid. At best the F group can be seen as neutral regarding exposure.

Week 0 : baseline comparisons

At week 0, completers (n = 44) did not differ significantly across the three groups (see Table 1). The three groups were balanced for sex, age, duration

TABLE1. Obsessive-compulsive disorders: 44 completers: baseline data

	Fluvoxamine + Anti-exposure (F) n = 13	Fluvoxamine + Exposure (Fe) n = 16	Placebo + Exposure (Pe) n = 15
Sex: M	2	8	6
F	11	8	9
Age	37 (10.8)	35 (8.7)	35.8 (11.5)
OCD duration/yrs	12.7 (11.6)	16.7 (11.4)	10.7 (9.3)
Andrews – life events	3.7 (2.2)	2.6 (1.7)	3.5 (1.7)
Negative Expectations			
Behaviour therapy	2.1 (1.9)	1.4 (1.6)	1.8 (1.2)
Pharmacotherapy	2.4 (1.8)	2.7 (1.5)	3 (1.6)
DSM–III: Multiple axis I diagnoses			
Major depression	1	3	2
Dysthymic disorder	5	4	4
Panic disorder	1	0	1
Generalized anxiety	1	0	1
Agor. with Pan. Att.	0	2	2
Agor. without Pan. Att.	0	1	0
Social Phobia	1	2	1
Simple Phobia	0	0	1
DSM-III: Axis II: personality			
Schizoid	0	1	0
Histrionic	0	1	0
Avoidant	0	1	0
Dependent	1	1	0
Atypical	0	1	0
Compulsive	12	11	15
DSM-III: Axis III: physical disorders	3	3	5
DSM-III: Axis IV: psychosocial stressors	3.46 (2.02)	3.12 (1.40)	3.26 (1.48)
DSM-III: Axis V : adaptive functioning	3.69 (1.31)	3.31 (1.57)	3.53 (1.59)

Frequency or mean (± Standard Deviation) Agor. with or without Pan. Att. = agoraphobia with or without panic attacks. No between-group statistically significant difference on any of the variables (5% level)

of obsessive-compulsive disorder, life events, negative expectations regarding exposure and fluvoxamine, various multiple DSM-III axis I diagnoses, DSM-III axis II (personality diagnoses), DSM-III axis III (physical illness), DSM-III axis IV (stress) and DSM-III axis V (adaptation). As many as 19 patients (43%) had depression (6 major and 13 dysthymic).

All the measures of depression and rituals were balanced across the three groups (see Table 2).

TABLE 2. Obsessive-compulsive disorders: depression and obsession-compulsions measures: mean (± standard deviation) Pre-test, post-test (n = 44) and follow-up (n = 37)

		Fluvoxamine + Anti-exposure (F) n = 13	Fluvoxamine + Exposure (Fe) n = 16	Placebo + Exposure (Pe) n = 15
HRSD (17 items)				
	Week 0	19.5 (5)	19.2 (6.9)	17.2 (4.7)
	Week 24	10.46(6.98)	9.12(6.03)	15.13(5.74)*
	Week 48	11.27(6.02)	10.71(6.27)	12.17(10.38)
Retardation				
	Week 0	12 (8.8)	12.8 (8.7)	8.4 (4.2)
	Week 24	7.1 (7.78)	6.8 (7.40)	7.66(6.04)
	Week 48	8.45(6.93)	6.29(5.38)	6.67(6.10)
MADRS				
	Week 0	23.2 (9.5)	24.8 (9.3)	22.4 (9.3)
	Week 24	13.00(9.29)	10.00(6.2)	17.00(9.6)*
	Week 48	14.18(7.31)	12.21(9.01)	14.42(11.97)
BDI (13 items)				
	Week 0	16.3 (7.8)	14.6 (7.6)	14.9 (9.3)
	Week 24	9.07(6.11)	7.00(6.38)	12.13(7.01)
	Week 48	9.09(6.73)	7.92(8.26)	10.9 (12.7)
Target rituals (self)				
Time	Week 0	23.1 (8.4)	20.6 (8.3)	23.4 (7.2)
	Week 24	11.69(7.85)	7.93(7.82)	15.33(8.59)
	Week 48	14.63(8.68)	10.42(9.27)	11.47(9.32)
Discomfort				
	Week 0	24.3 (7.8)	21.4 (7.7)	23.6 (6.1)
	Week 24	11.76(9.47)	9.37(7.86)	15.53(8.05)
	Week 48	13.09(8.43)	10.78(8.64)	13.33(15.41)
Duration per day				
	Week 0	6.8 (1.72)	1 (1.59)	6.5 (1.8)
	Week 24	3.61(2.72)	3.87(2.52)	5.20(2.30)
	Week 48	4.45(3.11)	4.07(3)	4.42(2.6)
Target rituals (assessor)				
Time	Week 0	24.8 (7.5)	23.3 (5.8)	25 (6.25)
	Week 24	12.84(7.78)	8.50(7.30)	15.60(9.2)
	Week 48	13.5 (3.11)	10.3 (8.7)	11.9 (9.7)
Discomfort				
	Week 0	25.7 (7)	24.7 (5.8)	27.6 (2.6)
	Week 24	11.30(10.27)	10.25(8.04)	17.00(8.35)
	Week 48	13.18(8.5)	12.21(9.25)	13.3 (9.8)

Duration per day

	Week 0	7 (1.6)	7.3 (1.1)	7.20 (1.3)
	Week 24	4.07 (2.56)	3.93 (2.26)	5.40 (2.19)
	Week 48	4.09 (2.59)	4 (2.80)	4.67 (2.27)
Behavioural avoidance test (BAT)				
Avoidance	Week 0	2.1 (1.71)	2.7 (1.3)	3 (1)
	Week 24	1.07 (1.03)	0.87 (0.88)	1.20 (1.20)
	Week 48	1.27 (1.27)	1.31 (1.32)	1.33 (1.15)
Discomfort				
	Week 0	22 (8.6)	22 (9.3)	27.7 (5.3)
	Week 24	11.46 (6.75)	9.12 (6.55)	15.61 (7.61)
	Week 48	13.8 (9)	10.7 (8.7)	14.1 (8.08)
Compulsive activity checklist (CAC)				
	Week 0	32.7 (18.1)	26 (12.6)	29.76 (21.3)
	Week 24	21.53 (12.56)	14.56 (17.38)	24.33 (18.36)
	Week 48	24.9 (17.8)	11.7 (11.5)	22.8 (14.9)

HRSD = Hamilton Rating Scale for Depression. MADRS = Montgomery Asberg Depression Rating Scale. BDI = Beck Depression Inventory (shorter 13 item form). At follow-up as one subject was not able to fill in BAT, BDI and CAC, calculations were made on 36 subjects for these three variables.
* Significant between group difference of the changes from week 0 to week 24 (p < .05)

Baseline comparability of the three groups was established for the same variables in the 50 patients re-evaluated at week 8 (see Table 3; complete data available upon request).

TABLE 3. Obsessive-compulsive disorders week 0 and week 8 (n = 50)

	Fluvoxamine + Anti-exposure (F) n = 15	Fluvoxamine + Exposure (Fe) n = 17	Placebo + Exposure (Pe) n = 18
Beck 13 items			
Week 0	16.00 (7.55)	15.76 (8.87)	17.00 (9.94)
Week 8	10.60 (6.17)	10.29 (7.69)	14.61 (8.45)
Target rituals (self)			
Time			
Week 0	21.73 (8.87)	20.52 (8.07)	23.05 (7.17)
Week 8	10.35 (7.22)	7.64 (6.58)	14.38 (8.91)
Discomfort			
Week 0	22.46 (8.76)	21.35 (7.48)	24.16 (5.95)
Week 8	7.21 (6.32)	8.41 (6.84)	15.11 (8.07)
Duration per day			
Week 0	6.66 (1.91)	7.05 (1.56)	6.55 (1.65)
Week 8	3.8 (2.32)	4.00 (2.44)	5.66 (2.24)*

Mean (± standard deviation)
* Significant between group difference (comparison of the change from pre-test to week 8, p < 0.05)

46

Results at Week 8 Early Outcomes (self-ratings only, see Table 3).

1. Within group change from week 0 to 8

    Within group changes were significant for Beck Depression Inventory and ritual duration per day in the two groups receiving Fluvoxamine ($p = 0.01$). There was a trend towards reduction of total rituals duration per day in the Exposure + Placebo group ($p = 0.05$), but this did not reach statistical significance. Ritual repetition and discomfort were significantly reduced in all three groups.

2. Between group comparison of the change from week 0 to 8

    A significant between group difference was found for total duration of rituals per day only ($p = 0.011$). The two groups receiving fluvoxamine were better than exposure with placebo ($p = 0.02$) (see Table 3).

3. Criterion of ritual improvement: global criterion of improvement

    The general criterion of improvement did not show any difference between the three groups: 5 patients were improved in the F group, compared with 3 in the Fe group, and 1 in the Pe group: Chi^2 (df 2) = 4.27, p = 0.11.

Results at Week 24

1. Within-group change

    The three groups showed a positive effect on rituals and depression, but the within group positive effect of combined treatment was a "broad spectrum" one.

    The F group showed a reduction in depression as rated by HRSD, MADRS and BDI but not on the retardation scale. Antiritualistic effects appeared on target rituals as evaluated by both self and assessor (time, discomfort and duration per day), as well as an effect on discomfort rated by the Behavioural Avoidance Test. Avoidance rated on the Behavioural Avoidance Test and the compulsion checklist showed only a trend ($p = 0.05$). Ten of the 13 measures changed significantly while 2 exhibited a trend towards significance.

    The Fe group showed a change in all the measures of depression and rituals ($p = 0.01$).

    The Pe group showed a more limited antidepressive effect which was demonstrated with MADRS only ($p = 0.01$). A trend towards significance was found on the Beck Depression Inventory ($p = 0.05$). A significant antiritualistic effect was seen on all the measures of rituals ($p = 0.01$) except for total duration of ritual per day (S); however, the total duration of ritual per day (A) showed a significant change ($p = 0.01$). Nine of the 13 measures changed significantly while 3 exhibited a trend towards significance.

2. Between-group comparison of the change from week 0 to 24.

    Significant between group differences were found for Hamilton depression scale ($p = 0.002$). Multiple paired comparisons showed that F gave equal results to Fe ($p < 0.10$) and both were better than Pe ($p = 0.02$). MADRS showed an overall significant difference ($p = 0.005$). Multiple comparisons found that Fe was superior to Pe (p = 0.002). Thus, F and Fe patients improved more on depression measures than Pe patients did. As there was a significant change on all the measures in the Fe group compared with 9 in the Pe group we tested the superiority of fluvoxamine against placebo using Hotelling T^2 on the 13 variables measuring both depression and rituals. The difference was highly statistically significant in favour of fluvoxamine:

$T^2 = 26.282$, F (df = 13) = 15.407, p < 0.0001.

3. Global criterion of improvement

    As far as completers were concerned there were no significant differences between the three groups. Seven patients (54%) in the F group, 11 in the Fe group (69%) and 6 in the Pe group (40%) were "successes": Chi^2 (df 2) = 2.51, NS. Including the drop-outs as failures did not modify the significance of the comparison: Chi^2 (df 2) = 2.91, NS.

    Follow-up: Results at Week 48

    Six months after the end of the treatment 9 patients were lost to follow-up in the F group, compared with 6 in the Fe group and 8 in the Pe group ($Chi^2 = 0.987$, p = 0.61). Five patients needed no treatment in the F group compared with 10 in the Fe group and 7 in the Pe group. One in the F group and 4 in the Pe group had new treatment. The same treatment was resumed in 5 patients in the F group, compared with 4 in the Fe group and 2 in the Pe group. The between group difference was non-significant: Chi^2 (df 4) = 6.09, p = 0.19.

1. Within group change

    No difference was found between weeks 24 and 48 on all the measures. Thus the gains obtained at week 24 were maintained in all three groups, six months after withdrawal of the treatments.

2. Between group comparison of the change from week 24 to 48

    No difference between the three treatment conditions appeared when the changes between week 24 and 48 were compared at this point (see Table 2).

3. Global criterion of improvement

    The general criterion of ritual improvement showed 5 successes in the F group (45%) compared with 9 (64%) in the Fe group and 6 (50%) in the Pe group: Chi^2 (df 2) = 0.99, p = 0.60.

Depression and Ritual Improvement at Week 24

The sample was fairly depressed to start with (mean and median = 19 on Hamilton depression scale). We tested some of the possible relationships noted by Marks.[4]

1. Does week 0 depression (Hamilton) correlate with level of rituals (total duration per day) at week 24?

    High levels of depression at pre-test did not predict fluvoxamine or exposure effect on rituals at post-test: In the F group: rho(11) = −0.22, NS. Only a trend appeared in the Fe group: rho(14) = −0.559, p = 0.05.

48

2. Does high versus low depression (Hamilton 19 as cut-off) at week 0 predict level of rituals (total duration per day) at week 24? Chi^2 using HRSD median score[19] as cut-off point and the criterion of ritual improvement were computed. All dropouts were counted as failures to allow statistical analysis. A trend appeared only in the Fe group (see Table 4).

TABLE 4. Baseline depression level and outcome at week 24 test

	Fluvoxamine + Anti-exposure (F) n = 20		Fluvoxamine + Exposure (Fe) n = 20		Placebo + Exposure (Pe) n = 20	
	Success	Failure	Success	Failure	Success	Failure
HRSD > = 19	5	5	4	8	2	7
HRSD < 19	2	8	7	1	4	7
(p)	0.34		0.054		0.49	

Chi^2 or Fisher test. Success: decrease in rituals during per day: more than 30%. All the dropouts are counted as failures.

3. Does pre-post reduction in Depression (Hamilton) correlate with pre-post reduction in total duration of rituals per day?

Spearman-rank correlation was computed for each of the three groups. A strong correlation appeared for the F group only: rho(11) = 0.88, p = 0.01. The Fe group rho(14) = 0.14, and the Pe group: rho(13) = 0.41 had lower and non-significant correlations. Thus baseline depression only weakly predicted outcome of rituals with fluvoxamine. Improvements in depression and rituals were related in the F group. Depression was unrelated to outcome in the Pe group.

DISCUSSION

FLUVOXAMINE and exposure results

On within group measures fluvoxamine and exposure were comparably anti-ritualistic at weeks 24 and 48. Between group effects were less impressive. When the F and Fe groups were compared, i.e. Fluvoxamine intake was comparable in both groups there was no significant difference between anti-exposure and exposure at any measurement point. When the Fe and Pe groups were compared i.e. exposure level was comparable, fluvoxamine had a significantly better effect than placebo on rituals at week 8 only, and on depression at week 24 (post-test). Antidepressive effects of exposure were comparable with those of fluvoxamine at weeks 8 and 48.

Our results accord with those of Price et al.[19], Perse et al.[20] and Goodman et al.[21] suggesting that fluvoxamine reduces both rituals and depression in the short term. They are also in line with the outcomes of Marks et al.[6] who found that clomipramine was more effective than placebo after 8 weeks of treatment. Moreover, they confirm the outcomes of Marks et al.[6,7] which in both these controlled studies showed that the significant superiority of clomipramine for improvement of rituals did not persist.

In our study no more relapses appeared at week 48, after fluvoxamine withdrawal in the F group than after cessation of behaviour therapy in the Pe group. However, the conclusions which can be drawn from the week 48 ratings are limited because they were obtained on less than half of the 20 patients originally randomised to each group (9 F, 9 Fe, 10 Pe). At a week 43 follow up, Marks et al.[6] found no difference between clomipramine plus exposure and placebo plus exposure. Clomipramine with antiexposure had been ineffective to week 18 after which antiexposure patients had insisted on other treatment as they had not improved, and so were crossed over to have exposure.

Our F patients complied very poorly with antiexposure instructions, while those of Marks et al.[6], who emphasized anti-exposure more strongly, complied well. Our patients had, on average, a substantially more depressed mood than those of Marks et al.[6]: (mean Hamilton 19, compared with 8), but were comparable with those of the Marks et al.[7] study (mean Hamilton = 18). In this early study clomipramine was effective only in depressed obsessive compulsives.

Benzodiazepine association

The effect on outcome of discontinuous use of bromazepam in about two-thirds of the subjects should be discussed: however, there is no evidence in the literature of any benzodiazepine effectiveness on rituals.[4]

Sample Size

Though our sample is larger than in most studies in this field our relatively small sample size may still increase the risk of type II errors. When the Fe group was compared with the F group the percentage of improved patients was slightly though non-significantly greater, at weeks 24 and 48, for combined treatment than where patients had only one or other treatment. Relapses were also less frequent with combined treatment: 5 of 9 F patients, 0 of 9 Fe patients, and 4 of 10 Pe patients who were rated at week 48 had had further treatment. Perhaps larger numbers would have yielded more significant results in favour of the combination of drug and psychological treatment. The statistical power of the comparisons of the changes between week 0 and week

24 was calculated for each of the 13 variables. For the comparison of Fe and Pe the statistical power of the depression rating scales comparisons ranged from 57 to 97%; statistical power for obsession-compulsions rating scales were less satisfying (3 to 54%). For the comparison F-Pe calculation was possible for Hamilton Depression Rating Scale (85%) only, but not for the other depression scale; for obsession-compulsions the range was 6 to 41%. For the comparison of Fe with F the statistical power of depression rating scales the range was 3-25% (table available upon request). This means that at least 35 patients per group were needed to show the superiority of Fe over Pe for rituals on the global criterion of improvement.

Obsessive-compulsive disorder, as represented in our sample, is a severe life-long illness which often requires chronic treatment; either behavioural or pharmacological. The combination of drug and behaviour therapy may have a better prophjylactic effecvt on relapses.

A larger scale and longer study is needed to answer this important question. However, in our study, the effect of fluvoxamine on rituals had disappeared at week 24, and its antidepressant effects at week 48. Therefore there is no indication that long-term treatment is beneficial for most patients, although some might benefit from such drugs given over years. Relapse is not a major problem after exposure as has been demonstrated in 2 to 6 year follow up studies.[22]

Fluvoxamine Action on Rituals

Only patients in the F group showed a highly significant correlation (0.88) between reduction in depression and outcome on rituals. This is consistent with another fluvoxamine study by Perse[21] who found that reduction in depression and in rituals correlated in depressed, but not in non-depressed obsessive compulsives. These two studies suggest that reduction of depression may play a role in fluvoxamine effects on rituals in depressed obsessive compulsive patients. However, reduction of anxiety and rituals by fluvoxamine treatment might produce a secondary reduction of depression. Patients with a low or high initial level of depression improved equally in the F group: absence of baseline depression, then, does not prevent the action of fluvoxamine on rituals in this group. It should be emphasised that baseline depression was quite accurate in predicting (0.054) a positive outcome at week 24 in the Fe group. No such relationship between depression and modification of rituals was found in the non-drug treatment group (Pe). Alternatively, fluvoxamine might be acting also on mechanisms upstream of both depression and rituals.

Acknowledgements

The pilot part of the study was supported by a grant from INSERM (PRC: 12007). Assessment tools validations were supported by a grant from "Les Hospices Civils de Lyon, Hospital Neurologique Pierre Wertheimer". The controlled part of the study was supported by grant from DUPHAR-FRANCE. We wish to thank Pr. J.P. Boissel for methodological advice, Annie Pascal-Duinat, Janine Guerin and Ouafae Achachi for therapeutic assistance and Martine Bessy for computer and statistical work.

REFERENCES

1 Thoren, R., Asberg, M., Cronholm, B., Jonertedt, L. and Traskman, L. Clomipramine treatment of obsessive-compulsive disorder: I. A controlled study. *Arch Gen Psychiatry* 1980;**37**:1281-1285.
2 Monteiro, W., Lelliott, P., Marks, I. and Noshirvani, H. Anorgasmia from clomipramine, in obsessive-compulsive disorder. *Br J Psychiatry* 1986;**151**:197-112.
3 Zohar, J. and Insel, T. Obsessive-compulsive disorder: psychobiological approaches to diagnosis, treatment and pathophysiology. *Biol Psychiatry* 1987;**22**:667-687.
4 Marks, I. "Fears, Phobias, and Rituals: Panic, Anxiety and their Disorders". *Oxford University Press, New York* 1987.
5 Flament, M., Rapoport, J., Berrg, C., Sceery, W., Kilts, C., Mellstrom, B. and Linnoila M. Clomipramine treatment of childhood obsessive-compulsive disorder. A double blind controlled study. *Arch Gen Psychiatry* 1985;**42**:977-983.
6 Marks, I., Lelliott, P., Basoglu, M., Nochirvani, H., Monteiro, H., Cohen, D. and Kasvikis, Y. Clomipramine, self-exposure and therapist aided exposure in obsessive-compulsive ritualisers. *Br J Psychiatry* 1988;**152**:522-534.
7 Marks, I., Stern, R.S., Mawson, D., Cobb, J. and McDonald, R. Clomipramine and exposure for obsessive-compulsive rituals: I. *Br J Psychiatry* 1980;**136**:1-25.
8 Mawson, D., Marks, I. and Ramm, L. Clomipramine and exposure for chronic obsessive-compulsive rituals III. Two year follow-up and further findings. *Br J Psychiatry* 1982;**140**:11-18.
9 Klock, C., Brower, G., Van Praag, H. and Doogan, D. Fluvoxamine and clomipramine in depressed patients. A double-blind clinical study. *Acta Psychiatr Scand* 1981;**64**:1-11.
10 Cottraux, J. Claustrat, B., Mollard, E. and Sluys, M. Depression and dexamethasone suppression test in 50 obsessive-compulsive patients. *J Anxiety Disord* 1989;**3**:7-13.
11 American Psychiatric Association. *Diagnostic and Statistical Manual, 3rd edition, A.P.A.*, Washington, DC 1980.
12 Foa, E. and Emmelkamp, P.M.G. *Failures in Behaviour Therapy.* Wiley, New York. 1983.
13 Marks, I., Hallam, R., Connoly, J. and Philpott, R. *Nursing in Behavioural Psychotherapy. An advanced Clinical Role for Nurses.* Whitefriars Press, London and Tonbridge. 1977.
14 Cottraux, J., Bouvard, M., Defayolle, M. and Messy, P. Validity and factorial structure study of the compulsive activity checklist. *Behav Ther* 1988;**19**:45-53.
15 Collet, L. and Cottraux, J. Inventaire abrege de la depression de Beck (13 items). Etude de la validite concurrente avec les echelles de Haqmilton et de ralentissement de Widlocher. *L'Encephale* 1986;**12**:77-79.
16 Widlocker, D. L'echelle de ralentissement depressif: fondements theoriques et premieres applications. *Psychol Med* 1981;**13**:53-60.
17 Montgomery, S. Clomipramine in obsessional neurosis: a placebo controlled trial. *Pharm Med* 1980;**1,2**:189-192.

18 Cottraux, J., Flachaire, E., Renaud, B. and Sluys, M. Dosage de la serontonine plaquettaire dans les obsessions-compulsions. *La Presse Med* 1987;**16,12**,590.

19 Price, L., Goodman, W., Charney, D., Rasmussen, S. and Heninger, G. Treatment of severe obsessive-compulsive disorder with Fluvoxamine. *Am J Psychiatry* 1987;**144,8**:1059-1061.

21 Goodman, W., Price, H., Rasmussen, S., Delgado, P., Heninger, G. and Charney, D. Efficacy of fluvoxamine in obsessive-compulsive disorder. A double-blind comparison with placebo. *Arch Gen Psychiatry* 1989; **46**:36-44.

22 O'Sullivan, G. and Marks, I. Long term follow-up of agoraphobia, panic, and obsessive-compulsive disorders. In: "Handbook of Anxiety" (Eds. R. Noyes *et al.*), vol 4, Elsevier, Amsterdam (in press). 1990.

THE EFFICACY OF SEROTONERGIC DRUGS IN OCD – POWER CALCULATIONS COMPARED WITH PLACEBO

Stuart A Montgomery, Naomi Fineberg and Deirdre B Montgomery

St Mary's Hospital Medical School, London

Assessing the efficacy of treatments in OCD

To establish the efficacy of a treatment in obsessional compulsive disorder (OCD) it is necessary to define the patients to be selected for study using internationally recognised diagnostic criteria. The criteria developed in DSMIII and DSMIIIR define a condition which is seen to produce moderate to severe impairment and which is relatively easy to distinguish from other conditions. These criteria have now been very widely adopted in efficacy studies.

A criticism which has been levelled at the DSMIII system is that the borderline between the illness OCD and obsessional worrying and anxiety is not clearly drawn. A number of individuals with OCD, during the course of the fluctuating illness, are found to fall into a subsyndromal category which may satisfy criteria for obsessive compulsive personality disorder. It is not clear in the DSMIII criteria whether these individuals should remain within the category of disorder. It would be logical, particularly with the development of effective pharmacotherapy, to recognise these individuals as suffering from OCD in partial remission. The whole question as to whether the subsyndromal category of obsessional disorder is really separate from OCD has not been properly settled. There are those who feel that as effective treatments are discovered it is likely that the syndrome of OCD will need to be more widely drawn and that a proportion of what is called obsessional personality disorder will turn out to be part of OCD proper and to benefit from these same treatments.

The design of studies in OCD

In all efficacy studies the severity scales on which the judgement of efficacy is to be based should be defined at the start of the study. The scales should be comprehensive and measure efficacy across the range of symptoms which represent the illness. Some of the studies in OCD were flawed by the inclusion of a large number of measures of individual symptoms or behaviours, and the selective reporting of those for which significant differences were found; the so-called fishing expedition. There are obvious statistical objections to this type of analysis, and if multiple scales are used, an appropriate adjustment of acceptable significance levels is required to demonstrate efficacy. Unfortunately the reports on some studies, more particularly those involving behaviour therapy, do not appear to take account of this requirement.

54

The efficacy scales currently most widely used in studies of OCD are the two scales derived from the Comprehensive Psychopathological Rating Scale,[1] a six item scale for those with pure OCD[2] and an eight item scale for OCD with concomitant depression.[3] The most widely used of the American scales is the Yale Brown scale for OCD.[4] All three of these scales have been validated by their ability to detect significant drug placebo differences in the conventional trial period. These scales have an advantage over some of the earlier instruments used in that they measure the effect on the severity of syndromally defined obsessional disorder rather than the effect on individual symptoms or behaviour. In avoiding the symptom list approach, bias towards particular kinds of obsessions and compulsions is avoided.

Conventionally the efficacy of antidepressant drugs is investigated in a four to six week trial period in depression. Although there is evidence that antidepressants will produce some further improvement in the treatment of depression from six to eight weeks, the dropouts for administrative and other reasons tend to compromise the ability of the longer studies to detect efficacy. The studies in OCD have consistently reported a signficant advantage for pharmacotherapy compared with placebo in the four to six week trial period and this has become accepted as the conventional trial period. Although it is possible to determine efficacy over shorter periods than four weeks the power of the study is weakened and there is a possible criticism that efficacy seen early may not be sustained. This is an important issue in view of the temporary improvement in anxiety symptoms which may be expected in the short term with some drugs such as the benzodiazepines. In this regard it is reassuring that with clomipramine there is evidence of longer term efficacy. The two large studies of de Veaugh Geiss et al[5] showed efficacy compared with placebo at ten weeks, and two studies have demonstrated efficacy compared with placebo at six months.

Unequivocal demonstration of efficacy requires a comparison against placebo. Such studies should of course be conducted under double blind controlled conditions and the customary design is a parallel group comparison, although it is possible for a crossover design to be used, provided that treatment order is random and carry over effects are taken into account. The analysis of response is normally undertaken using an analysis of variance with the initial severity as coveriant. Categorical response analysis is sometimes undertaken as well, although there are no generally agreed criteria for defining a responder. Since some of the treatments offered, including both behaviour therapy and clomipramine, have an appreciable dropout rate, it is necessary to undertake an intention to treat analysis including all those who have entered the first day of the clinical trial, in order to take account of the bias of only looking at the results with completers who tend, of course, to be responders.

The minimum size of study comparing two active treatments

There is now sufficient evidence to regard clomipramine as effective as an anti-obessional treatment. It is certainly the treatment, whether behavioural or pharmacotherapeutic, with the best efficacy data. If clomipramine were taken as the reference treatment it is possible to make some power calculations about the size of the studies necessary to demonstrate equal efficacy. There are several different formulae which may be used; that which is presented here is easily applied and understood,[6] where P is the expected response rate and F is

$$\frac{2 \times P \times 100 - P \times F \,(\text{alpha beta})}{10^2}$$

6.9 if one assumes that new antiobsessional treatment can be considered effective if it can be demonstrated with 95% confidence (alpha 0.05) that it is at worst 10% inferior to clomipramine accepting a 20% risk of missing a difference (beta 0.2).

If one takes the response rate of 65% reported for clomipramine in an early study[7] of non-depressed OCD patients the required number of patients in each treatment group works out at 360. This means that it is not possible to demonstrate equal efficacy in a study of less than 720 evaluable patients. If the response rate drops to 45% as reported in De Veaugh Geiss study[5] then the necessary minimum numbers rise to 784. Studies of this size are very difficult to achieve and exceed the total number of patients included in all of the controlled studies of OCD which have yet been published.

The size of studies compared with placebo

The assumptions which underlie the calculation of establishing a difference between placebo and an effective treatment are altogether more favourable in terms of the numbers needed.

$$= \frac{P_1 \times (100 - P_1) + P_2 \times (100 - P_2) \times F \,(\text{alpha beta})}{(P_2 - P_1)^2}$$

where P_1 is the expected placebo response (5%) and P_2 is the expected treatment response (65%) and F is the function of alpha and beta.[7] Assuming for example that alpha is 0.05 and beta is 0.1. F = 10.5 and only 8 – 9 patients would be required in each treatment group. These calculations demonstrate why it is possible for small studies to consistently show that a treatment is more effective than placebo. If the response rate drops to 60% the numbers required per treatment group only rises to 10 per group. If the response rate drops to 45% the numbers required rise to 20 per group. For all practical and ethical purposes therefore it is only possible to demonstrate that a treatment is effective if it is compared under appropriate double blind conditions with placebo or a neutral control.

Efficacy of 5-HT uptake inhibitors in pure OCD

There were suggestions in early open reports that clomipramine might have an effect on obsessional symptoms within depression. Obsessional symptoms do occur in depressed patients and it was difficult to know whether this response was part of the effect of an antidepressant in depressed patients or whether it might be a more specific effect.

In order to test whether clomipramine had a specific antiobsessional effect it was necessary to examine its efficacy in a group of pure OCD patients namely those without primary or significant secondary depression. In the first study to address the specificity of the antiobsessional effect of clomipramine[7] patients who were concomitantly depressed were excluded. The study used a crossover design with random order allocation to treatment for four weeks, with placebo and a low dose of 75mg clomipramine to protect blindness. The efficacy of clomipramine was shown, both in the crossover part of the design, and in the group comparison of clomipramine and placebo, in the first four weeks of the study. Clomipramine appeared to have an early onset of action with a significant difference compared with placebo emerging at 1, 3 and 4 weeks in the group comparison, despite this being a small study of 14 patients. In the crossover analysis a significant difference was observed at weeks 2, 3 and 4 weeks.

The most surprising aspect of this result was that a highly significant advantage could be detected for clomipramine in such a small number of patients. In retrospect, this was probably due to a combination of the strong antiobsessional effect of clomipramine and the very low placebo response rate. An important finding of this kind requires replication but it was 1989 before two large multicentre studies in OCD patients without concomitant depression also reported efficacy for clomipramine, with a significant difference from placebo detected at one to two weeks and increasing drug placebo difference apparent in a linear fashion for the duration of the ten week study.[5] Further replication was reported by Marks et al[8] in a small study which demonstrated the efficacy of clomipramine, despite the concomitant use of behaviour therapy in the placebo treated group. These results provide compelling evidence for the efficacy of clomipramine in pure OCD, and the results of the de Veaugh Geiss et al[5] formed the basis for the registration of the drug in the United States for this indication. (Table 1)

5-HT uptake inhibitors in OCD with depression

OCD frequently coexists with depressive symptoms: in the ECA study for example the co-occurrence of OCD and major depression both defined according to DSMIII criteria was reported to occur more than would be expected by chance with an odds ratio of 10.8 compared with the null value of 1.0.[9,10] On the surface it is possible of course that clomipramine's antidepressant effects may contribute to the efficacy of clomipramine in patients with OCD with depressive symptoms.

TABLE 1. Placebo controlled studies of clomipramine (CMI) in OCD without concomitant depression

Study	Design	Signif Diff
Montgomery[7] n = 14	Crossover CMI 75mg vs placebo	CMI > placebo (4 weeks)
Marks et al[8] n = 25 12	CMI 127-157mg+expos vs placebo+exposure	CMI > placebo (8 weeks)
de Veaugh Geiss et al[5] n = 122 119	CMI 100-300mg vs placebo	CMI > placebo (2-10 weeks)
n = 72 71	CMI 100-300mg vs placebo	CMI > placebo (2-10 weeks)

The evidence for the efficacy of clomipramine in OCD patients with varying degrees of depression was reported in five studies.[3,11,12,13,14] (Table 2) These studies were again rather small but a significant advantage for clomipramine compared with placebo was consistent. The power of these small studies to detect significant differences suggests that the effect comes principally from the antiobsessional effect of clomipramine rather than the antidepressant effect which would have required a much larger number of patients.

TABLE 2. Placebo controlled studies of clomipramine in OCD – concomitant depression not excluded

Study	Design	Signif Diff
Thoren et al[3] n = 8 8	CMI 150mg vs placebo	CMI > placebo (5 weeks)
Marks et al[11] n = 20 20	CMI 183mg vs placebo	CMI > placebo (4 weeks)
Insel et al[12] n = 12	crossover CMI 100-300mg vs placebo	CMI > placebo (4-6 weeks)
Flament et al[13] n = 19	crossover CMI 141mg vs placebo in children	CMI > placebo (5 weeks)
Mavissakalian et al[14] n = 7 5	CMI 100-300mg vs placebo	CMI > placebo (12 weeks)

Clomipramine is a potent 5-HT uptake inhibitor although it has an active metabolite with strong noradrenergic properties. While it seemed possible that the effect of clomipramine in OCD might be attributed to its serotonergic effect, the question could not be answered because of these noradrenergic properties. A more selective 5-HT uptake inhibitor, fluvoxamine, has however also been bound to be effective in OCD compared with placebo.[15,16,17] (Table 3) Both drugs are potent 5-HT uptake inhibitors and the evidence points to their efficacy being related to this pharmacological property.

TABLE 3. Selective 5HT reuptake inhibitors in OCD – Placebo controlled studies

Study	Design	OCD improvement
Fluvoxamine		
Price et al[30] n = 10	Placebo 2/52 then Fluvox 4/52 (single blind)	Fluvox > placebo (4 weeks)
Perse et al[16] n = 16	Crossover	Fluvox > placebo (8 weeks)
Goodman et al[15] n = 21 Flvx n = 21 Plac	Parallel	Fluvox > placebo (2 weeks)
Cottraux et al[17] n = 16 Flvx n = 15 Plac	Parallel Flvx + exposure vs Placebo + exposure	Fluvox > placebo (6 months)

Non-serotonergic antidepressants appear ineffective

The evidence in favour of other antidepressants without potent serotonergic properties is poor. In the first crossover study comparing clomipramine with desipramine, which is marred by the lack of control of treatment order effect, the response to desipramine was not significantly different from placebo, whereas a significant improved response was seen with clomipramine in the comparison.[18] In the second crossover study, which compared clomipramine directly with desipramine, the failure of desipramine was even more clearly seen.[19] Likewise, in the studies which included a comparison with imipramine, clomipramine was found to be superior at 6 and 12 weeks.[20] Foa et al[21] reported that imipramine did not have anti-obsessional effects though it appeared to have some antidepressant response effect. In the small three-way study by Thoren et al,[3] which compared clomipramine with nortriptyline and placebo, there was a significant effect for clomipramine, but nortriptyline appeared no different from placebo, and in a small study by Ananth et al,[22] which compared clomipramine with amitriptyline, there was a significant different from placebo in the clomipramine-treated group but not in the amitriptyline-treated group.

A significant difference between active treatments is not normally expected unless very large numbers are included in studies. The studies in OCD that have compared two antidepressants have been very small and yet an apparent superiority of clomipramine emerges which suggests that the reference TCAs are associated with little, if any, efficacy.

Monoamine oxidase inhibitors (MAOI), benzodiazepines and neuroleptics appear to be relatively ineffective.[12,23,24,25] This may reflect the fact that the studies were not carried out with as careful a methodology as they might have been but it does suggest that these drugs, which are known to have an effect on anxiety disorders or anxiety symptoms, are not effective in OCD.

Behaviour Therapy and OCD

The place of behaviour therapy in the treatment of OCD has come under increasing scrutiny as alternative therapies which are easier to use have been shown to have consistent and unequivocal efficacy. It is also clear in the efficacy studies that 5-HT uptake inhibitors are effective even in those centres which provided what was thought to be effective behaviour therapy to both placebo and the drug treated groups.[11,3,16] One would have expected that if behaviour therapy was effective it should have removed the significant difference in response between drug and placebo. The fact that it did not suggests that the behaviour therapy used in these centres was not as effective as drugs.

A serious reappraisal of the efficacy of behaviour therapy is made difficult by the lack of adequate short-term controlled studies, and the absence of medium and long term studies. The small numbers of short term efficacy studies reported, suffer from serious methodological flaws and are often inadequately, and consequently misleadingly, reported. A casual observer may think there are more independent studies than there really are, as some of the reports included patients from earlier studies rather than being new samples. For example, the study reported by Marks et at[26] includes the patients from the studies of Rachman et al,[27,28,29] with a small number of extra patients added.

The studies are small in size and have a treatment duration of between two and three weeks. There are no studies comparing behaviour therapy against a neutral control for a period longer than three weeks, and this is too short to make a proper assessment of efficacy. In these studies the treatment order is not random between relaxation therapy, the controls, and behaviour therapy, and the assessments are single blind on some tests only. In the three week study of Marks et all[11] no group difference is reported between placebo and behaviour therapy, only a comparison against an individual group base line. The small study of Marks et al[2] compares exposure therapy with antiexposure therapy which is not a neutral control. It is not possible to determine whether the difference reported can be attributed to a deterioration reported in the antiexposure group, or to improvement in the exposure group. (Table 4)

The evidence of efficacy overall is therefore weak, and there have been insufficient studies which were able to properly test the efficacy of behaviour therapy. The methodology necessary to undertake such studies has been worked out, and it should prove relatively easy to test efficacy of behaviour therapy to the same standards as those we expect for any treatment. It is a pity to leave a doubt unnecessarily over a treatment which may be shown in adequate testing to demonstrate efficacy.

TABLE 4. Behaviour therapy compared with neutral control

Single blind on some assessments

Author	Design	Result
Marks et al[26] includes Rachman et al[27,28] Hodgson et al[29]	Relaxation then exposure Not random n = 15 vs 20 Duration 3 weeks	? efficacy
Roper et al[31]	Exposure then relaxation then exposure n = 5 vs 5 vs 10 Duration 2 – 3 weeks	? efficacy
Marks et al[11]	Exposure plus placebo vs relax plus placebo n = 10 vs 10 Duration 3 weeks	No group difference reported ? efficacy

CONCLUSION

The clinical results from placebo controlled studies showing that potent 5-HT uptake inhibitors are effective in OCD, and that conventional and effective antidepressants, without direct potent effects on serotonin, are ineffective in OCD, remain the pivotal finding. The recognition that response in OCD is low or absent on placebo, and that effective drugs work in pure OCD without depression as well as in OCD with concomitant depression, argues for the separation of OCD as a distinct disorder. The balance of the clinical evidence argues for a separate identity for OCD and suggests that OCD may be a more directly serotonergic illness than depression. On the available evidence of efficacy the treatment of choice should be the 5-HT uptake inhibitors with behavioural therapy relegated to adjunct or second time treatment.

REFERENCES

1 Asberg M, Montgomery S A, Perris C, Schalling D, Sedvall G. A comprehensive psychopathological rating scale. Acta Psychiatr Scand 1978;Supp:271.
2 Montgomery S A and Montgomery D B. Measurement of change in psychiatric illness: new obsessional, schizophrenia and depression scales. Postgrad Med J 1980;supp 1:50–52.
3 Thoren P, Asberg M, Cronholm B, et al. Clomipramine Treatment and Obsessive Compulsive Disorder. Arch Gen Psyhiatry, 3 1980;37:1281–85.
4 Goodman W K, Price L H, Rasmussen S A et al. The Yale Brown Obsessive Compulsive Scale I: Development, use and reliability. Arch Gen Psychiatry 1989;46:1006–1011.
5 de Veaugh Geiss J, Landau P, Katz R. Treatment of obsessive compulsive disorder with clomipramine. Psychiatr Ann 198919:97–101.
6 Pocock S J. Clinical Trials a Practical Approach. John Wiley Chichester, 1983.
7 Montgomery S A. Clomipramine in Obsessional Neurosis: A placebo-controlled trial. Pharm Med 1980;1:(2), 189–192.

8 Marks I M, Lelliott P, Basoglu M *et al.* Clomipramine, Self-exposure and Therapist-aided Exposure for Obsessive-Compulsive Rituals. *Br J Psychiatry* 1988;**152**:522–534.

9 Burke J D, Regier D A, Christie K A. Epidemiology of Depression: recent findings from the NIMH epidermiologic catchment area programme. In: Depression and Anxiety. ed J A Swinkels. W Blijleven, Medidact Houten. 1988.

10 Boyd J H, Burke J D, Gruenberg E, *et al.* Exclusion criteria DSMIII. *Arch Gen Psychiatry* 1984;**41**:983–989.

11 Marks I M, Stern R S, Mawson D, Cobb J and McDonald R. Clomipramine and exposure for obsessive compulsive rituals: I. *Br J Psychiatry* 1980;**136**:1–25.

12 Insesl T R, Murphy D L, Cohen R M *et al:* Obsessive Compulsive Disorder – a double blind trial of clomipramine and clorgyline. *Arch Gen Psychiatry* 1983;**40**:605–612.

13 Flament M, Rapoport J, Berg C *et al.* Clomipramine Treatment of Childhood Obsessive Compulsive Disorder. *Arch Gen Psychiatry* 1985;**42**:977–983.

14 Mavikassalian M, Turner S, Michelson *et al.* Tricyclic Antidepressants in Obsessive-Compulsive Disorder: antiobsessional or antidepressant agents? *Am J Psychiatry* 1985;**142**:(5), 572–576.

15 Goodman W K, Price L H, Rasmussen S A *et al.* Efficacy of Fluvoxamine in obsessive compulsive disorder. *Arch Gen Psychiatry* 1989;**46**:36–44.

16 Perse T L, Greist J H, Jefferson J W *et al.* Fluvoxamine Treatment of Obsessive Compulsive Disorder. *Am J Psychiatry* 1987;**144**:1543–1548.

17 Cottraux J, Mollard E, Bouvard M *et al.* A controlled Study of Fluvoxamine and Exposure in Obsessive Compulsive Disorders. *Int Clin Psychopharmacol* 1990;**5**:17–30.

18 Insel T R, Mueller E A, Alterman I *et al.* Obsessive Compulsive Disorder and Serotonin: is there a connection? *Biol Psychiatry* 1985;**20**:1174–1188.

19 Leonard H, Swedo S, Rapoport J *et al.* Treatment of childhood obsessive compulsive disorder with clomipramine and desmethylimipramine: a double blind crossover comparison. *Psychopharmacol Bull* 1988;**24**:(1), 93–95.

20 Volavka J, Neziroglu F, Yaryura-Tobias J.A. Clomipramine and imipramine in obsessive-compulsive disorder. *Psyhiatr Res* 1985;**14**:85–93.

21 Foa E B, Steketee G, Kozak M J. *et al.* Imipramine and placebo in the treatment of obsessive compulsives: their effect on depression and on obsessional symptoms. *Psychopharmacol Bull* 1987;**23**:(1), 8–11.

22 Ananth J, Pecknold J L, Van den Steen N. *et al.* Double blind comparative study of clomipramine and amitriptyline in obsessive neurosis. *Prog neuro-psychopharmacol* 1981;**5**:257–262.

23 Orvin G H. Treatment of the phobic obsessive-compulsive patient with oxazepam, an improved benzodiazepine compound. *Psychosom* 1967;**8**:278–280.

24 Rao A V. A controlled trial with "Valium" in obsessive compulsive states. *J Indian Med Assoc* 1964;**42**:564–567.

25 Trethowan J W H & Scott P A L. Chlorpromazine in obsessive-compulsive and allied disorders. *Lancet* 1955:781–785.

26 Marks I M, Hodgson R, Rachman S. Treatment of chronic obsessive-compulsive neurosis by in-vivo exposure. *Br J Psychiatry* 1975;**127**:349–364.

27 Rachman S, Hodgson R, Marks I M. Treatment of chronic obsessive-compulsive neurosis. *Behav Res Ther* 1971;**9**:237–247.

28 Rachman S, Marks I M, Hodgson R. The treatment of obsessive-compulsive neurotics by modelling and flooding in vivo. *Behav Res Ther* 1973;**11**:463–471.

29 Hodgson R, Rachman S, Marks I M. The treatment of obsessive-compulsive neurosis: follow up on further findings. *Behav Res Ther* 1972;**10**:181–189.

30 Price L H, Goodman W K, Charney D S, *et al.* Treatment of severe obsessive-compulsive disorder with fluvoxamine. *Am J Psychiatry* 1987;**144**:1059–1061.

31 Roper R, Rachman S, Marks I M. Passive and participant modelling in exposure treatment of obsessive compulsive disorder. *Behav Res Ther* **1975;13**:271–279.

FLUVOXAMINE IN THE TREATMENT OF OBSESSIVE COMPULSIVE DISORDER

Wayne K Goodman

Yale University School of Medicine, Connecticut U.S.A.

In recent years, there have been major advances int he pharmacotherapy of Obsessive Compulsive Disorder (OCD). For example, a number of double-blind studies have shown that the potent serotonin (5-hydroxytryptamine; 5-HT) reuptake inhibitor clomipramine is more effective than placebo in the treatment of OCD.[1,2,3,4,5,6,7,8] Moreover, in recent double-blind trials in OCD outpatients, clomipramine was significantly superior to the relatively selective norepinephrine reuptake inhibitor desipramine.[9,10] Together, these drug response data lend support to the hypothesis that the acute 5-HT reuptake properties of an antidepressant drug are relevant to its efficacy as an anti-obsessive-compulsive agent. However, because a major metabolite of clomipramine is a potent blocker of norepinephrine reuptake, it is unclear whether the efficacy of clomipramine in OCD is related solely to its effects on 5-HT transport.

In recent years, trials have been conducted in OCD patients with a newer generation of antidepressants which are both potent and selective blockers of 5-HT reuptake (e.g., fluvoxamine, zimelidine, sertraline, venlafaxine, and fluoxetine). Unlike clomipramine, none of these medications loses its selectivity for blocking 5-HT reuptake in vivo.[11] Also, in contrast to tricyclics like clomipramine, these drugs lack significant affinity for cholinergic, alpha-adrenergic, serotonergic, and histaminic receptors. This may explain the relatively lower incidence of anticholinergic and cardiovascular side effects and sedation with the newer agents. Recent studies suggest that this class of drugs may provide new options in the treatment of OCD as well as, furnish clues to its pathophysiology. The Role of fluvoxamine in the treatment of OCD is the subject of the present chapter.

Fluvoxamine was originally developed in Europe as an antidepressant. In most published double-blind trials in depressed patients, fluvoxamine has been shown to be significantly better than placebo and equal in efficacy to tricyclics such as imipramine and clomipramine.[12] On the basis of its monoamine reuptake blocking properties, several groups have conducted trials of fluvoxamine in patients with OCD.[13]

REVIEW OF STUDIES OF FLUVOXAMINE IN OCD

In a single-blind study of fluvoxamine, six of ten inpatients with severe OCD were "responders" on the basis of a clinical rating of "much" or "very much improved" on a modified version of the Clinical Global Impressions (CGI)[14] scale. On this conservative measure of clinical outcome, patients rated as "somewhat improved" were classified as "nonresponders". Most of the patients in this study were previously refractory to adequate trials of other antidepressant medications. These encouraging findings are further supported by two double-blind studies of fluvoxamine in outpatients with OCD.

In a study conducted at the University of Wisconsin, 16 OCD patients completed a 20-week randomised crossover trial which compared fluvoxamine with placebo.[15] Patients received active fluvoxamine treatment for eight weeks. There was a two-week single-blind placebo period prior to the start of treatment, and between treatments (wash-out period). Fluvoxamine was found to be effective on several different measures of OCD. For example, marked clinical improvement in OCD was only associated with the active drug phase, with 9 of 16 (56%) patients classified as "better" during fluvoxamine treatment.

Similar findings were obtained in a parallel group design study conducted jointly at Yale and Brown.[16] Forty-two OCD patients were randomly assigned to 6 to 8 weeks of treatment with either fluvoxamine (up to 300 mg daily) or placebo. Patients received supportive psychotherapy and were encouraged to "resist" their obsessive-compulsive symptoms. All patients had a principal diagnosis of OCD (according to DSM-III), but approximately one-half the sample had coexisting major depression. Weekly assessment of severity of OCD and depression was based on semi-structured patient and clinician ratings. The principal outcome measure for OCD in this study, and several other recent studies, was the Yale-Brown Obsessive Compulsive Scale (Y-BOCS). This 10-item clinician-rated instrument was developed as a specific measure of the severity of obsessive-compulsive symptoms.[16] Unlike some other rating instruments intended for use in OCD, the total score on the Y-BOCS is independent of the type or number of obsessive-compulsive symptoms that are present. The ratings on the first five items on the Y-BOCS reflect the composite effect of the patient's obsessive symptoms on five dimensions of severity: time occupied, distress, interference, resistance, and control; the second five items assess the net effect of the patient's compulsive symptoms on five parallel-constructed measures of severity. Each item on the Y-BOCS is rated on a 5-point scale from 0 = "no symptoms" to 4 = "extreme symptoms", so that the range of the total score (sum of items 1 to 10) = 0 to 40. The reliability, validity, and sensitivity to change of the Y-BOCS have been established in formal studies of its psychometric properties.[17,18]

In this controlled trial, fluvoxamine was found superior to placebo on four different measures of OCD, including the Y-BOCS.[16] On the basis of mean Y-BOCS scores, analysis of variance with repeated measures revealed significant changes from baseline beginning at week two of fluvoxamine treatment. In contrast, there were no significant changes in mean total Y-BOCS scores for any week following baseline in the placebo-treated group. Similarly, analysis of response category data showed that fluvoxamine was effective in reducing the severity of obsessive-compulsive symptoms. In the fluvoxamine-treated group, nine of 21 patients were responders (as defined above according to CGI scores), whereas none of the 21 placebo-treated patients were rated as responders. This remarkably low placebo response rate seems characteristic of outpatient OCD studies and contrasts with a much higher placebo rate typically seen in drug trials in depressed outpatients.

Antidepressant or Antiobessional?

The design of this study also allowed us to examine whether the anti-obsessive-compulusive effects of fluvoxamine could be differentiated from its antidepressant action. Patients with a range of severity in secondary depressive symptoms were entered into the study and rating instruments were selected to optimise separation of response of obsessive-compulsive vs. response of depressive symptoms. The Y-BOCS, in particular, lends itself to examination of selective changes in obsessive-compulsive symptoms since it was constructed to exclude items concerning severity of depressive symptoms. Analysis of the relationship between measures of improvement in OCD (including the Y-BOCS) and measures of depression disclosed that the anti-obsessive-compulsive effects of fluvoxamine were independent of baseline levels of depression.[13] For example, there was no significant correlation between fluvoxamine-induced improvement in Y-BOCS scores and baseline ratings of depression (based on the Hamilton Rating Scale for depression (HAM-D).[19] If fluvoxamine was primarily acting as an antidepressant, then OCD patients with concurrent major depression might be predicted to have the best response. This was not the case in this study. Of the nine responders to fluvoxamine, three were classified at initial presentation as depressed but six were nondepressed. In fact, according to baseline HAM-D ratings, the most depressed and the least depressed OCD patient were both rated as responders to fluvoxamine treatment.

The University of Wisconsin group had similar findings for the relationships between the antidepressant and anti-obsessive-compulsive responses to fluvoxamine. Perse and her colleagues found that improvement in obsessive-compulsive symptoms was unrelated to severity of depression at baseline. This experience with fluvoxamine in OCD mirrors that of most studies which have attempted to distinguish the anti-obsessive-compulsive from the antidepressant actions of other antidepressants in OCD.[20] In all but one study of clomipramine in OCD,[3] coexisting depression was not a prerequisite to an anti-obsessive-compulsive response.[1,8] Multicentre, double-blind, placebo-controlled trials of fluvoxamine in non-depressed OCD outpatients have recently been concluded in North America, but the results are not yet available.

66

Magnitude and Time Course of Clinical Response

Although, in our outpatient study, we found statistically significant mean group effects of fluvoxamine on obsessive-compulsive symptoms after only two weeks of treatment, clinically meaningful changes were generally not apparent until at least 4-6 weeks of treatment.[13,16] In fact, of seven patients that were considered only partial responders by week 6, five converted to full responders after two additional weeks of fluvoxamine at week 8. Also, mean total Y-BOCS scores for the fluvoxamine-treated group continued to decrease throughout the trial. Mean Y-BOCS scores were decreased 25% from baseline at 8 weeks compared with 20% from baseline at 6 weeks of fluvoxamine treatment. Thus, it appears with fluvoxamine, and perhaps with other antidepressants in OCD, that at least 8 weeks may be needed for an adequate treatment trial.

In the nine fluvoxamine responders, the mean Y-BOCS scores at the conclusion of treatment were 42% below baseline ratings. This degree of improvement represented major gains in social and vocational functioning. The mean Y-BOCS score of this responder group at the end of the trial was 14 ± 7 ($\pm$SD), which corresponds with a global severity in the mild to moderate range. Thus, these patients were much improved but not entirely free of symptoms. In fact, no patient had a Y-BOCS score of 0 at the end of the double-blind trial. Similar results have been obtained for clomipramine in OCD with respect to rate and degree of treatment response.[2,8]

A COMPARISON OF FLUVOXAMINE VS. DESIPRAMINE IN OCD

To further examine whether the serotonergic actions of fluvoxamine are relevant to its anti-obsessive-compulsive efficacy, fluvoxamine was compared with the relatively selective norepinephrine reuptake inhibitor desipramine in 40 outpatients with OCD. After one week of single-blind placebo, the patients were randomised to 8 weeks of double-blind treatment with fluvoxamine or desipramine. Medication dosage was increased to a maximum of 300 mg daily as tolerated. OCD patients with depression were not excluded provided OCD was judged the principal diagnosis. There were no significant differences in the clinical characteristics of the fluvoxamine (n=21; mean age=39 ± 10; M=7, F=14) and desipramine (n=19; mean age=37 ± 14; M=12, F=7) treatment groups, although there tended to be more males in the desipramine group, and, conversely, more females in the fluvoxamine group. As measured by reduction in total Y-BOCS scores, fluvoxamine was found to be superior to desipramine in the treatment of OCD (F=4.09; df=7, 266; p<0.001). Eleven of 21 (52%) patients treated with fluvoxamine for 8 weeks were responders compared with 2 of 19 (11%) who received desipramine for eight weeks (p<0.01, Fisher's exact probability test). The percentage decrease in total Y-BOCS score from baseline among responders to fluvoxamine was 45% (final Y-BOCS = 15.5 ± 7). Analysis of the separate effects of treatment on HAM-D scores showed that fluvoxamine, but not desipramine, was effective in reducing depressive symptoms in patients with OCD. In "responders" to fluvoxamine (n=11), the mean HAM-D score at the end of the trial was 7.3±5, representing a 65% decrease from baseline. There was no significant correlation between baseline HAM-D ratings and changes from baseline in Y-BOCS ratings at week 8 (r=0.27, p=0.23).

These findings provide additional evidence that the acute 5-HT reuptake properties of a medication are relevant to its anti-obsessive-compulsive efficacy and complement previous studies showing that the potent but non-selective 5-HT reuptake inhibitor clomipramine is also more effective than desipramine.[9,10]

IMPLICATIONS OF DRUG RESPONSE DATA FOR THE NEUROBIOLOGY OF OCD

The efficacy studies reviewed here suggest that fluvoxamine possesses clini-cally significant anti-obsessive-compulsive properties. These findings also support the hypothesis that potency of 5-HT reuptake inhibition may be critical to the anti-obsessive-compulsive efficacy of a drug. However, since significant 5-HT reuptake inhibition is achieved after a single dose of a 5-HT reuptake inhibitor, yet a therapeutic response usually requires weeks of drug treatment, other mechanisms may be responsible for the anti-obsessive-compulsive action of fluvoxamine. One possibility is that fluvoxamine-induced adaptive changes in 5-HT autorecepter sensitivity, which takes several weeks to develop, may be more directly related to anti-obsessive-compulsive efficacy.[21] Alternatively, although several lines of preclinical and clinical evidence suggest that chronic 5-HT reuptake inhibitor administration does have important effects on brain 5-HT function (e.g., increased 5-HT transmis-sion in electrophysiological studies,[21] there is preclinical evidence that other monoaminergic systems may be indirectly affected by chronic fluvoxamine. For example, in laboratory animals, chronic administration of fluvoxamine has been associated with down-regulation of beta-adrenergic receptors.[22] There is also ample preclinical evidence for important anatomical and functional inter-actions between serotonergic and dopaminergic systems.[23] Hence, it is conceivable that chronic fluvoxamine treatment induces compensatory alter-ations in other neurochemical systems which are more directly tied to the reduction of obsessive-compulsive symptoms. Future clinical studies are needed to assess the effects of chronic fluvoxamine treatment on brain monoamine function.

GUIDELINES TO USE OF FLUVOXAMINE IN OCD

Choice of Antidepressant

In general, the choice of a drug treatment depends on consideration of its relative efficacy, side effects (safety), and availability. As reviewed here and elsewhere, there is considerable published evidence that clomipramine is effective in OCD.[8] Fewer data are available on fluoxetine, yet recent open-label studies[24,25] and clinical experience suggest it is also beneficial in OCD. As discussed herein, several studies support the superiority of fluvoxamine over placebo. A recent study also demonstrated that fluvoxamine was more effective than desipramine in the treatment of OCD.[26] The relative anti-obsessive-compulsive efficacy of fluvoxamine to other potent 5-HT reuptake blockers, such as clomipramine or fluoxetine, has not been directly studied. On the other hand, comparison of response rates across independent placebo-controlled studies suggest that fluvoxamine and clomipramine are roughly equivalent. Because of the recent availability of fluoxetine in the USA, we have attempted to substitute fluoxetine for fluvoxamine in some OCD patients chronically maintained and improved on fluvoxamine. In more cases, we have been successful in making this change without apparent loss of efficacy. However, because these changes were conducted in an open fashion, and without the benefit of a placebo control, it is impossible to draw firm conclusions about comparative efficacy.

In our hands, the most commonly reported side effects for fluvoxamine, in order of decreasing frequency, are daytime drowsiness, nausea, insomnia, headache, tremors, and delayed orgasm. Nausea, tremor, and sexual dysfunction (particularly delayed or absent orgasm) seem to be common side effects of all the potent 5-HT reuptake inhibitors. Most patients on fluvoxamine, and other 5-HT reuptake inhibitors, develop tolerance to nausea. If nausea is severe it may be necessary to maintain the patient at the lowest possible daily dose until signs of tolerance develop. Unlike many other antidepressants, fluoxetine does not seem to induce weight gain and, in some cases, may actually result in weight loss.[14] Studies are needed to determine whether this effect on weight is sustained during long-term use. Our own experience suggests that, in some OCD patients, appetite and weight may increase moderately after approximately six months of treatment with either fluoxetine or fluvoxamine (Goodman et al., unpublished data). However, in evaluating these possible late side effects, it is difficult to separate direct pharmacological actions from the secondary effects of reduced obsessive-compulsive symptoms and improved mood on appetite and eating habits. Also based on our anecdotal experience, we have observed that the side effect profiles of fluvoxamine and fluoxetine are different in some respects, with fluvoxamine producing more sedation, and fluoxetine causing more insomnia (Goodman et al, unpublished data). In general, there are less side effects with fluvoxamine and fluoxetine than with clomipramine. The side effect profile of clomipramine includes symptoms typical of both potent 5-HT reuptake inhibitors (e.g., nausea and delayed orgasm) and tricyclics. Anticholinergic side effects (e.g., dry mouth, constipation, urinary retention), orthostatic hypotension, sedation, and weight gain are common with clomipramine and other tricyclics.

The seizure incidence of clomipramine has been reported to be somewhat higher than other tricyclics.[27] However, recent studies by the manufacturer suggest that the risk of seizures associated with clomipramine may be dose-related, with the majority occurring above 250 mg daily. Rash and systemic signs of drug sensitivity (e.g., fever, arthralgias, oedema, carpal tunnel

69

syndrome) have been reported by approximately 4% of patients receiving fluoxetine. Reversible elevations in liver transaminases have been reported with fluvoxamine, fluoxetine, and clomipramine.

In the UK, fluvoxamine fluoxetine and clomipramine are all available on a general presecription basis; in the USA, fluvoxamine is still investigational. At the time of this writing, fluoxetine, which is approved for depression, is the only potent and select 5-HT reuptake inhibitor widely available in the USA. Zimelidine was withdrawn from clinical testing because of adverse neurological events. Several other potent and selective 5-HT reuptake inhibitors, including sertraline and venlafaxine, are currently undergoing testing in the treatment of OCD.

Adequacy of Trial

A working definition of an adequate drug trial includes parameters for duration of treatment, dose, and bioavailability (e.g., a reliable measure of the drug level actually attained in plasma or brain). For the treatment of depression, an adequate antidepressant trial is usually four to six weeks; in the treatment of OCD, a minimum of six, and as many as ten to twelve weeks of 5-HT reuptake inhibitor treatment may be required. Fluvoxamine is prescribed up to a maximum daily dose of 300 mg, as tolerated; however, there are presently no published data on the relationship between fluvoxamine dose (or plasma levels) and clinical outcome in OCD. To encourage compliance, it is useful to educate the patient regarding the expected time-course and magnitude of response to fluvoxamine.

When assessing outcome, it is important to differentiate response of depressive and obsessive-compulsive symptoms. Clear identification of the target obsessive-compulsive symptoms is critical to this assessment. Weekly administration of a structured rating instrument for OCD, such as the Y-BOCS ,[16] should facilitate monitoring of clinical response to treatment.

THE TREATMENT REFRACTORY PATIENT

There have been few controlled evaluations of pharmacological approaches to OCD patients who have not responded to an adequate trial of a 5-HT reuptake inhibitor alone. For example, it is unclear whether the first step in the treatment algorithm should involve a trial with another 5-HT reuptake inhibitor or an augmentation strategy. In the clinic at Yale, there are examples of individual OCD patients who had failed trials with two 5-HT reuptake inhibitors (e.g., clomipramine and fluoxetine), and then had a robust response to a third 5-HT reuptake inhibitor (e.g., fluvoxamine), in all three possible permutations. Although a systematic evaluation of this approach is needed, in clinical practice, it seems justified to try fluvoxamine in OCD patients who have failed trials with other 5-HT reuptake inhibitors.

In depressed patients, one approach to treating nonresponders or partial responders has been to add lithium (which may augment 5-HT function[28] to antidepressant drug treatment. Some OCD patients may improve when lithium is added to chronic treatment with potent 5-HT reuptake inhibitors (e.g., clomipramine[29,30] or fluvoxamine[31]), but this strategy seems generally less effective in OCD than it is in depression. Addition of tryptophan, the amino acid precursor of 5-HT, has been reported helpful in an OCD patient on clomipramine,[29] but ineffective in OCD patients on trazodone.[32] Large supplements of tryptophan are contraindicated in patients on fluoxetine because of reports of neurological side effects with this combination.[33] In an open case series, some OCD patients seemed to benefit from the addition of low doses of antipsychotic medication to fluvoxamine treatment.[34] More detailed studies of antidepressant-antipsychotic combination therapy are needed in OCD.

SUMMARY

On the basis of four published studies, the potent and selective 5-HT reuptake inhibitor fluvoxamine is an effective treatment for OCD. At least eight, and as many as twelve, weeks of treatment may be required for an adequate trial. Response to the anti-obsessive-compulsive effects of fluvoxamine is independent of severity of depression at baseline. More than 50% of patients with OCD are significantly improved after a trial with fluvoxamine. These findings are roughly comparable with the rate of improvement shown in similar studies with clomipramine treatment of OCD, the current gold standard for anti-obsessive-compulsive drug treatment. Despite the success of fluvoxamine and other potent 5-HT reuptake inhibitors in OCD, not all patients benefit from this treatment. One possible explanation for this finding is that OCD is heterogeneous, and that only certain subtypes of OCD may be responsive to treatment with 5-HT reuptake inhibitors alone.

In contrast to the treatment of depression, the addition of lithium to ongoing 5-HT reuptake inhibitor therapy is usually ineffective in treatment-refractory OCD. It is evident that new and more effective pharmacological strategies are needed for the treatment-refractory OCD patient. Combination therapy with a potent 5-HT reuptake inhibitor and dopamine antagonist (e.g., pimozide) shows promise, but the appropriate target population needs to be better defined, especially before long-term treatment is considered. A detailed discussion of behavior therapy is beyond the scope of this discussion, but there is reason to believe that the combination of a 5-HT reuptake inhibitor and behavior therapy is presently the most effective treatment of OCD. Until reliable predictors of outcome are identified or studies have been conducted in which the anti-obsessive-compulsive efficacy of the different 5-HT reuptake inhibitors can be compared directly, the initial choice of a medication treatment for an individual patient with OCD may be based mostly on its side effects profile and availability.

ACKNOWLEDGEMENT

Studies of fluvoxamine were supported in part by NIMH grants MH-25642, MH-30929, and MH-40140 and by the State of Connecticut. Fluvoxamine was generously provided by Reid-Rowell, Incl., Marietta, GA. The authors thank the research, clinical, and clerical staffs of the Clinical Neuroscience Research Unit for their assistance and Betsy Kyle who typed the manuscript.

REFERENCES

1 Montgomery S A. Clomipramine in Obsessional Neurosis: A placebo-controlled trial. *Pharm Med* 1980;**1**(2), 189–192.

2 Thorén P, Asberg M, Cronholm B, Jornestedt L, Träskman L. Clomipramine treatment of obsessive-compulsive disorder. I. A controlled clinical trial. *Arch Gen Psychiatry* 1980;**37**:1281–1285.

3 Marks I M, Stern R S, Mawson D, Cobb J, McDonald B. Clomipramine and exposure for obsessive compulsive rituals. *Br J Psychiatry* 1980;**136**:1–25.

4 Insel T R, Murphy D L, Cohen R M *et al.* Obsessive Compulsive Disorder – a double blind trial of clomipramine and clorgyline. *Arch Gen Psychiatry* 1983;**40**:605–612.

5 Flament M, Rapoport J, Berg C *et al.* Clomipramine Treatment of childhood obsessive compulsive disorder. *Arch Gen Psychiatry* 1985;**42**:977–983.

6 Mavikassalian M, Turner S, Michelson *et al.* Tricyclic antidepressants in obsessive-compulsive disorder: antiobsessional or antidepressant agents? *Am J Psychiatry* 1985;**142**:(5), 572–576.

7 Marks I M, Lelliott P, Basoglu M *et al.* clomipramine, self-exposure and therapist-aided exposure for obsessive-compulsive rituals. *Br J Psychiatry* 1988;**152**:522–534.

8 DeVeaugh-Geiss J, Landau P, Katz R. Treatment of obsessive compulsive disorder with clomipramine. *Psychiatr Ann* 1989;**19**:97–101.

9 Leonard H, Swedo S, Rapoport J L, Coffey M, Cheslow D. Treatment of childhood obsessive compulsive disorder with clomipramine and desmethylimipramine: A double-blind crossover comparison. *Psychopharmacol Bull* 1988;**24**:93–95.

10 Zohar J, Insel T R. Obsessive-compulsive disorder: Psychobiological approaches to diagnosis, treatment and pathophysiology. *Biol Psychiatry* 1987;**22**:667–687.

11 Fuller R W, Wong D T. Serotonin reuptake blockers in vitro and in vivo. *J Clin Psychopharmacol* 1987;**7**:36S–43S.

12 Benfield P, Ward A. Fluvoxamine. A review of its pharmacodynamic and pharmacokinetic properties, and therapeutic efficacy in depressive illness. *Drugs* 1986; **32**:313–334.

13 Goodman W K, Price L H, Charney D S. Fluvoxamine in obsessive compulsive disorder. *Psychiatr Ann* 1989;**19**:92–96.

14 Price L H, Goodman W K, Charney D S *et al.* Treatment of severe obsessive-disorder with fluvoxamine. *Am J Psychiatry* 1987;**144**:1059–1061.

15 Perse T L, Greist J H, Jefferson J W *et al.* Fluvoxamine treatment of obsessive disorder. *Am J Psychiatry* 1988;**144**:1543–1548.

16 Goodman W K, Price L H, Rasmussen S A, Delgado P L, Heninger G R, Charney D S. Efficacy of fluvoxamine in obsessive-compulsive disorder. A double-blind comparison with placebo. *Arch Gen Psychiatry* 1985;**46**:36–44.

72

17 Goodman W K, Price L H, Rasmussen S A, Mazure C, Fleischmann R, Hill C, Heninger G R, Charney D S. The Yale-Brown Obsessive Compulsive Scale (Y-BOCS): Part I. Development, use and reliability. *Arch Gen Psychiatry* 1989; **46**:1006–1011.

18 Goodman W K, Price L H, Rasmussen S A, Mazure C, Delgado P, Heninger G R Charney D S. The yale-brown obsessive compulsive scale (Y-BOCS): Part II. validity. *Arch Gen Psychiatry* 1989;**46**:1012–1016.

19 Hamilton M. Development of a rating scale for primary depressive illness. *Br J Soc Clin Psychol* 1967;**6**:278–296.

20 Insel T R, Zohar J. 1987. Psychopharmacologic approaches to obsessive-compulsive disorder. In: Meltzer H Y eds. Psychopharmacology: The Third Generation of Progress, pp 1205–1210. Raven Press: New York.

21 Blier P, deMontigny C, Chaput Y. Modifications of the serotonin system by anti-depressant treatments: Implications for the therapeutic response in major depression. *J Clin Psychopharmacol* 1987;**7**:24S–35S.

22 Bradford L D, Schipper J. Biochemical effects in rats after long term treatment with fluvoxamine and clovoxamine: Postsynaptic changes. Pro Soc Neurosci Annu Meet, Dallas, Texas. *Abstract 224.6* 1985.

23 Crespi F, Martin K F, Marsden C. Simultaneous in vivo voltammetric measurement of striatal extracellular DOPAC and 5-HIAA levels: effect of electrical stimulation of DA and 5HT neuronal pathways. *Neurosci Lett* 1988;**90**:285–291.

24 Jenike M A, Buttolph L, Baer L, Ricciardi J, Holland A. Open trial of fluoxetine in obsessive-compulsive disorder. *Am J Psychiatry* 1989;**146**:909–911.

25 Liebowitz M R, Hollander E, Schneier F *et al.* Fluoxetine treatment of obsessive-compulsive disorder: An open clinical trial. *J Clin Psychopharmacol* 1989;**9**: 423–427.

26 Goodman W K, Price L H, Delgado P L, Palumbo J, Krystal J H, Nagy L M, Rasmussen S A, Heninger G R, Charney D S. Specificity of serotonin reuptake inhibitors in the treatment of obsessive compulsive disorder: Comparison of fluvoxamine and desipramine. *Arch Gen Psychiatry* June, 1990.

27 Anonymous. Clomipramine for obsessive compulsive disorder. *Med Lett* 1988;**30**: 45–47.

28 Blier P, deMontigny C. Short-term lithium administration enhances serotonergic neurotransmission electrophysiological evidence in the rat CNS. *Eur J Pharmacol* 1985;**113**:69–79.

29 Rasmussen S A. Lithium and tryptophan augmentation in clomipramine-resistant obsessive-compulsive disorder. *Am J Psychiatry* 1984;**141**:1283–1285.

30 Eisenberg J, Asnis G. Lithium as an adjunct treatment in obsessive-compulsive disorder. *Am J Psychiatry* 1985;**142**:663.

31 McDougle C J, Price L H, Goodman W K, Charney D S, Heninger G R. Lithium augmentation in fluvoxamine-refractory obsessive compulsive disorder. *Amer Psychiatr Assoc New Res.* Abstract #302.

32 Mattes J A. A pilot study of combined trazodone and tryptophan in obsessive-compulsive disorder. *Int Clin Psychopharmacol* 1986;**1**:170–173.

33 Steiner W, Fontaine R. Toxic reaction following the combined administration of fluvoxamine and l-tryptophan: Five case reports. *Biol Psychiatry* 1967;**21**:1067–1071.

34 McDougle C J, Goodman W K, Price L H, Delgado P L, Krystal J H, Charney D S, Heninger G R. Neuroleptic addition in fluvoxamine-refractory OCD. *Amer Psychiatr Assoc New Res Abstracts* #NR350.

OBSESSIONAL DISORDER AND THE GILLES DE LA TOURETTE SYNDROME

Mary M Robertson

University College & Middlesex Schools of Medicine

The Gilles de la Tourette Syndrome (GTS) is a movement disorder character-ised by both multiple motor and one or more vocal tics which usually occur many times a day, in bouts. The anatomical location, number, frequency, com-plexity and severity of the tics change over time and characteristically the onset of the disorder is before the age of 21 years.[1]

The first clear medical description of GTS was made in 1825, when Itard[2] reported the case of the then 26 year old Marquise de Dampierre, a French noblewomen, who had developed symptoms of GTS at the age of seven and who, because of the socially unacceptable nature of her vocalisations, was compelled to live as a recluse until she died at the age of 85. Of note is that she also manifested symptoms of obsessive-compulsive disorder (OCD) in addition to a tic disorder. A convincing case has been made[3,4] that the 18th century liter-ary figure Dr Samuel Johnson suffered from GTS. Miss Lucy Porter told James Boswell[5] that when Dr Johnson "was introduced to her mother, his appearance was very forbidding;...he often had, seemingly, convulsive starts and odd gesticulations, which tended at once surprise and ridicule". He apparently had a wide repertoire of motor tics such as mouth opening, lip pursing, eye squinting, and perpetual convulsive movements of the hands and feet. He had vocalisations including "ejaculations of the Lord's prayer", whistling sounds, sounds like the clucking of a hen and of a whale exhaling.[5,3,4] He also exhibited echolalia and mild self-injurious behaviour, and it has also been suggested that Dr Johnson suffered from severe OCD in addition to his motor and vocal tics. He felt impelled to measure his footsteps, perform complex gestures when he crossed a threshold and involuntarily touch specific objects.[4]

The exact prevalence of GTS is unknown, but a currently accepted figure is 0.5 per thousand (approximately 110,000 patients in the USA and 27,500 in the United Kingdom,[6] but even this may prove to be an underestimate. Recent studies[7,8,9] suggest that many cases of GTS are mild, do not come to medical attention and do not require pharmacological treatment.

GTS is found in all cultures and racial groups, but it is rare among the American black population. Most large cohorts of patients with GTS have come from the USA, but substantial numbers of patients have also been reported from the Soviet Union, the United Kingdom, Japan, Gemany, the Netherlands, Denmark and China. These studies, plus case reports from all parts of the world highlight the worldwide distribution of the disorder. GTS occurs three or four times more commonly in males than in females, and it is found in all social classes.[10]

The clinical characteristics of patients with GTS appear to be independent of culture, as they occur with some degree of uniformity irrespective of the country of origin. The age of onset of GTS symptoms ranges from two to 15 years with a mean of seven years being commonly reported. The most frequent initial symptoms are tics involving the eyes (such as eye blinking), head nodding and facial grimacing which are also the most common tics. GTS is often referred to as a tic disorder, but patients with GTS usually exhibit a wide variety of complicated movements including touching, hitting, jumping, smelling of the hands or objects, spitting, kicking, stamping, squatting and a variety of complexities of gait.[10]

The onset of vocalisations is usually later than that of the motor tics, with a mean age of 11 years, and grunting, coughing, throat-clearing, barking, snorting, explosive utterances, screaming, humming, hissing, clicking, colloquial emotional exclamations and inarticulate sounds are the usual utterances. Coprolalia (the involuntary inappropriate uttering of obscenities) is reported in approximately one third of patients and usually has a mean age of onset of 14 years. Copropraxia (the involuntary and inappropriate making of obscene gestures) is reported in 3% – 21% of GTS patients. Echolalia (the imitation of sounds or words) and echopraxia (imitation of actions) occur in 11% – 44% of patients. Tics and vocalisations are characteristically aggravated by anxiety, stress, boredom, fatigue and excitement, while sleep, alcohol, orgasm, fever, relaxation or concentration lead to temporary disappearance of symptoms.[10]

Many types of behaviour have been reported to occur frequently in patients with GTS. Some types of behaviour, such as obsessive-compulsive disorder are intimately linked to GTS (see below) and are thus probably an integral part of the syndrome, whereas others such as hyperactivity, attention deficit disorder and learning difficulties occur in a substantial number of patients (30% – 60%) and are probably often the symptoms for which the patient is referred to the physician.[10] Antisocial behaviour, inappropriate sexual activity, exhibitionism, aggressive behaviour and discipline problems [10] and self-injury[11] are found in a substantial percentage of clinic GTS populations. From the author's experience in clincial,[12] family and pedigree[9] settings, and from the data of epidemiological surveys,[8] it is suggested that relatively few GTS subjects in the community exhibit antisocial behaviour, and that the excess reporting of such behaviours may well reflect an artefact of selective referrals, and thus represent ascertainment bias.[10]

Electroencephalogram (EEG) abnormalities have been found in 12% to 37% of patient cohorts: abnormalities are non-specific and there is no evidence of any paroxysmal activity time-locked to the tics.[10] Complementing the wide spectrum of clinical manifestations of GTS is an equally wide variety in EEG patterns.[10] Evoked potentials have been studied in patients with GTS, but no consistent abnormalities have been demonstrated.[10]

Robertson et al[12] documented 71 out of 73 patients with GTS as having normal CT scans and the abnormality in both cases was cavum septum pellucidum. Other studies have noted CT scan abnormalities in 16 GTS patients. In other words only 18 out of 172 documented CT scans have been abnormal, and the abnormalities do not appear to be of direct aetiological significance.[10] In addition, the vast majority of normal scans suggest that the pathology in GTS is not structural. Only one group has used brain imaging studies to investigate function in GTS.[13,14] In the first controlled study a PET scan (using an ECAT 11 scanner and fluorine-18-labelled fluorodeoxyglucose) showed abnormalities in five GTS patients.[13] In the GTS patients there was a relatively close positive association between metabolism in the basal ganglia (particularly the corpus striatum) and metabolism throughout the cerebral cortex. In addition the cortical regions in which glucose metabolism had a close inverse association with the severity of vocal tics, clustered in the middle and inferior parts of both frontal lobes, and extended posteriorly from the frontal poles to the post central gyrus. Coprolalia, in contrast, was inversely correlated with hypometabolism in the left parasylvian region.[13] Continuing their work in the area, Chase et al[14] assessed 12 untreated GTS patients and compared them with matched normal controls using the improved NINCDS NEURO PET scanner with a higher resolution and sensitivity than the ECAT 11 scanner: at horizontal levels from 8.4-8.8 cm caudal to the vertex, non-normalised glucose utilisation rates were approximately 15% below control values in the frontal cingulate and insular cortex, and the inferior corpus striatum ($p - 0.01$). Chase et al[14] also evaluated two males (21 and 40 years) and one female (28 years) with GTS using magnetic resonance imaging with a 0.5 Tesla Picker International scanner or a 1.5 Tesla General Electric Sigma scanner, and no definite abnormalities were detected. Post-mortem studies have not revealed any consistent abnormalities.[15,16,17] Robertson et al[18] reported that ten out of 80 GTS patients had an abnormally low serum copper level. Two of the ten were investigated in detail with copper radioisotope studies and both exhibited abnormalities of copper metabolism.

The aetiology of GTS is unknown, but it has been suggested that it is inherited as an autosomal dominant with incomplete penetrance.[9,10] The pathogenesis is also unknown but it is thought that dopamine is implicated, as dopamine antagonists are useful in treatment of symptoms in the majority of patients with GTS. In addition the pathophysiology of GTS may be located in the basal ganglia.[10]

It is perhaps no coincidence that some of the first comments on the association between GTS and OCD were made by Gilles de La Tourette himself in 1889,[19] when he noted the anxieties and phobias of his patients. In that paper he noted the ideas of Guinon[20] who suggested that "tiqueurs" nearly always had associated psychiatric disorders characterised by multiple phobias, arithmomania and agoraphobia. Grasset[21] also referred to the obsessions and phobias of patients, which were to him an accompaniment of the tic disorder, representing psychical tics. Thereafter, Meige and Feindel,[22] in "confessions of a victim to tic", describe a patient whom they consider to be the prototype of a tic patient. In retrospect, it is clear that this patient would now be diagnosed as having GTS. He had motor tics which began at the age of eleven years, echophenomena (copying behaviours), a "tic of phonation dating back to his 15th year" and "an impulse to use slang". In addition he was impulsive, had suicidal tendencies and had obsessive-compulsive behaviour. Meige and Feindel[22] state: "the frequency with which obsessions, or at least a proclivity for them, and tics are associated, cannot be a simple coincidence". They describe case histories of patients with typical features of OCD including the relief of anxiety that accompanied the carrying out of a particular motor act. However, in addition to the close link between the motor movement and a compulsion, they noted that often there was no direct connection between a patient's obsessions and the tics, the former occurring in the form of extraordinary scrupulousness, phobias and excessive punctiliousness in their actions. They specifically mentioned arithmomania, onomatomania (the dread of uttering a forbidden word or the impulse to intercollate another) and *folie du pourquoi*, which is the irresistible habit of seeking explanations for the most commonplace facts by asking perpetual questions. Kinnear-Wilson,[23] the neurologist, also acknowledged a relationship between tics and OCD: "no feature is more prominent in tics than its irresistibility......The element of compulsion links the condition intimately to the vast group of obsessions and fixed ideas". Ascher[24] noted that all of the five GTS patients he reported had obsessive personalities, while Bockner[25] commented that the majority of GTS cases described in the literature had obsessive-compulsive neurosis.

There is a growing literature in modern scientific writings on the relationship between OCD and GTS, and it is becoming increasingly evident that there is a clear and strong association between the two disorders.[10] To date eleven studies have documented GTS patients as having obsessional symptoms, traits or illness, in significant percentages of patient populations: 11%,[26] 31%,[27] 32%,[28] 33%,[29] 38%,[30] and as high as 60%,[31] 66%,[32] 68%,[33] 71%,[34] 74%,[35] and 80%.[36] Moreover, in controlled studies[37-40] GTS patients were found to have higher scores on obsessive-compulsive inventories and to show more obsessive-compulsive behaviours than normal controls. The scores and behaviour ratings were as high as those of patients with OCD. Robertson *et al*[12] found that 37% of clinic GTS patients have obsessive compulsive behaviours and, using standardised rating scales, found much higher scores in GTS patients compared with normative data. In addition, coprolalia and echophenomena were significantly associated with obsessive – compulsive phenomena.[12] The argument for a strong association between GTS and OCD also comes from both pedigree[41,7,42,43,40,9] and epidemiological[8] studies which suggest that not only do patients with mild GTS have significant obsessive-compulsive behaviours, but also that OCD may well be a phenotype of the anticipated GTS gene. It is therefore of added interest that in the GTS twin study of Jenkins and Ashby,[44] both twins were described as obsessional.

One may also examine the association from the perspective of OCD patients, and Rapoport[45] notes that about 20% of OCD patients have tics. Serotonin is the neuro-transmitter most implicated in the pathogenesis of OCD.[45] Non-specific frontal neuroradiological abnormalities have been documented in OCD.[46,47] It has been suggested[48,49,50] that OCD, at least in some patients, may be due to basal ganglia dysfunction, while other findings support evidence of involvement of the caudate nucleus.[51] One study showed that in OCD metabolic rates were significantly increased bilaterally in the caudate nucleus and hypermetabolism in the orbitofrontal cortex.[52] Further evidence for the link comes from the writings by Williams *et al*[53] who described a patient with a compulsive movement disorder with cavitation of the caudate nucleus and Pitman and Jenike[54] who describe a patient with OCD and coprolalia. Further evidence for the organic aetiology of OCD comes from the fact that there are studies indicating that genetic factors may be important in the aetiology of OCD.[55-64] Further work in the area is needed to know the exact genetic mechanism involved in OCD, and whether OCD is related genetically and phenomenologically to GTS.

In conclusion, therefore, it would appear that at least some types of obsessional disorder are an integral part of GTS, and, in this context it is interesting to note that Pierre Janet in 1903, in his treatise *Les Obsessions et la Psychasthenie*, described three stages of psychasthenic illness: the first was the "psychasthenic state", the second "forced agitations", which included motor tics, while the third was obsessions and compulsions.[65]

REFERENCES

1 American Psychiatric Association. Diagnostic and Statistical Manual of Mental Disorders (3rd edn, revised) (DSM-III-R). Washington DC: American Psychiatric Association.

2 Itard J M G. Memoire sur quelques fonctions involuntaires des appareils de la locomotion de la prehension et de la voix. *Arch Gen Med* 1825;**8**:385–407.

3 McHenry L C Jr. Samuel Johnson's tics and gesticulations. *J Hist Med* 1967;**22**:152–168.

4 Murray T J. Dr Samuel Johnson's movement disorders. *Br Med J*, 1979;**i**:1610–1614.

5 Boswell J. The Life of Samuel Johnson LLD. London: George Routledge & Sons. 1867.

6 Bruun R. Gilles de la Tourette's syndrome: an overview of clinical experience. *J Am Acad Child Psychiatry* 1984;**23**:126–133.

7 Kurlan R, Behr J, Medved L *et al*. Severity of Tourette's syndrome in one large kindred: implication for determination of disease prevalence rate. *Neurology* 1987;**44**:268–269.

8 Caine E D, McBride M C, Chiverton P *et al*. Tourette syndrome in Monroe county school children. *Neurology* 1988;**38**:472–475.

9 Robertson M M and Gourdie A. Familial Tourette's syndrome in a large British pedigree: Associated psychopathology, severity of tourette's and potential for linkage analysis. *Br J Psychiatry* 1990;**156**:515–521.

10 Robertson M M. The Gilles de la Tourette syndrome: The current status. *Br J Psychiatry* 1989;**154**:147–169.

11 Robertson M M, Trimble M R, Lees A J. Self-injurious behaviour and the Gilles de la Tourette syndrome. A clinical study and review of the literature. *Psychol Med* 1989;**19**:611–625.

12 Robertson M M, Trimble M R, Lees A J. The psychopathology of the Gilles de la Tourette syndrome: a phenomenological analysis. *Br J Psychiatry* 1988;**152**:383–389.

13 Chase T N, Foster N L, Fedio P, *et al*. Gilles de la Tourette syndrome: studies with the fluorine-18-labelled fluorodeoxyglucose positron emission tomographic method. *Ann Neurol* 1984;**15**:(Suppl), S175.

14 Chase T N, Geoffrey V, Gillespie M, *et al.* Structural and functional studies of Gilles de la Tourette syndrome. *Rev Neurol (Paris)* 1986;**142**:851–855.

15 Dewulf A and Van Bogaert L. Etudes anatomo-cliniques de syndromes hyper-cinetiques complexes – partie 3. Une observation anatomo-clinique de maladie des tics (Gilles de la Tourette). *Monatsschr Psychiatr Neurol* 1941;**104**:53–61.

16 Balthasar K. Uber das anatomische substrat der generalisierten tic-krankheit (maladie des tics, Gilles de la Tourette): Entwicklungshemmung des corpus striatum. *Arch Psychiatr Nervenkr (Berlin)* 1957;**195**: 531–549.

17 Haber S N, Kowall N W, Vonsattel J P *et al.* Gilles de la Tourette's syndrome: a postmortem neuropathological and immunohistochemical study. *J Neurol Sci* 1986;**75**:225–241.

18 Robertson M, Evans K, Robins A, *et al.* Abnormalities of copper in Gilles de la Tourette syndrome. *Biol Psychiatry* 1987;**22**:968–978.

19 Gilles de la Tourette G. La maladie des tics convulsifs. *La Sem Med* 1899;**19**:153–156.

20 Guinon G. Sur la maladie des tics convulsifs. *Rev Med* 1886;**6**:50–80.

21 Grasset J. Lecons sur un cas de maladie des tics et un cas de tremblement singulier de la tete et des membres gauches. *Arch Neurol* 1890;**20**:27–45, 187–211.

22 Meige H and Feindel E. Tics and Their Treatment. Translated and edited by SAK Wilson, New York: William Wood and Company. 1907

23 Wilson SAK. Tics and child conditions. *J Neurol Psychopathol* 1927;**8**:93–109.

24 Ascher E. Psychodynamic considerations in Gilles de la Tourette's disease (maladie des tics): with a report of five cases and discussion of the literature. *Am J Psychiatry* 1948;**105**:267–276.

25 Bockner S. Gilles de la Tourette's disease. *J Ment Sci* 1959;**105**:1078–1081.

26 Kelman D H. Gilles de la Tourette's disease in children: a review of the literature. *J Child Psychol Psychiatry* 1965;**6**:219–226.

27 Fernando S J M. Gilles de la Tourette's syndrome: a report on four cases and a review of published case reports. *Brit J Psychiatry* 1967;**113**:607–617.

28 Comings D E and Comings B G. Tourette syndrome: Clinical and psychological aspects of 250 cases. *Am J Hum Gen* 1985;**37**:435–450.

29 Abuzzahab F E and Anderson F O. Gilles de la Tourette's syndrome. *Minnesote Med* 1973;**56**:492–496.

30 Asam U. A follow-up study of Tourette syndrome. In: A J Friedhoff and T N Chase, eds. Gilles de la Tourette syndrome. Advances in Neurology, Vol 35, New York, Raven Press. 1982.

31 Hagin R A, Beecher R, Pagano G *et al.* Effects of Tourette syndrome on learning. In: A J Friedhoff and T N Chase, eds. Gilles de la Tourette syndrome. Advances in Neurology, Vol 35, New York, Raven Press. 1982.

32 Montgomery M A, Clayton P J and Friedhoff A J. Psychiatric illness in Tourette syndrome patients and first-degree relatives. In: Gilles de la Tourette Syndrome (eds A J Friedhoff and T N Chase) Advances in Neurology, Vol 35, New York, Raven Press. 1982.

33 Nee L E, Caine E D, Polinsky R J *et al.* Gilles de la Tourette syndrome: clinical and family study of 50 cases. *Ann Neurol* 1980;**7**:41–49.

34 Morphew J A and Sim M. Gilles de la Tourette's syndrome: a clinical and psychopathological study. *Br J Med Psychol* 1969;**42**:293–301.

35 Stefl M E. Mental health needs associated with Tourette syndrome. *Am J Pub Health* 1984;**74**:1310–1313.

36 Yaryura-Tobias J A, Nezirogulu F, Foward S *et al.* Clinical aspects of Gilles de la Tourette syndrom. *J Orthomolec Psychiatry* 1981;**10**:263–268.
37 Frankel M, Cummings J L, Robertson M M *et al.* Obsessions and compulsions in Gilles de la Tourette's syndrome. *Neurology* 1986;**36**:378–382.
38 Green R C and Pitman R K. Tourette syndrome and obsessive-compulsive disorder. In: M A Kenike, L Baer & W O Minichiello eds. Obsessive-Compulsive Disorders: Theory and Management. Littleton MA: PSGP Publishing Co. 1986.
39 Van de Wetering B J M, Cohen A P, Minderaa R B *et al.* Het Syndroom van Gilles de la Tourette: Klinische Bevindigen. *Ned Tijdschr Geneeskd* 1988;**132**:21–25.
40 Comings D E and Comings B G. A controlled study of Tourette syndrome, 1 – VII. *Am J Hum Gen* 1987;**41**:701–866.
41 Kurlan R, Behr J, Medved L *et al.* Familial Tourette's syndrome: report of a large pedigree and potential for linkage analysis. *Neurology* 1986;**36**:772–776.
42 Pauls D L, Leckman J, Towbin K E, *et al.* A possible genetic relationship exists between Tourette's syndrome and obsessive-compulsive disorder. *Psychopharm Bull* 1986a;**22**:730–733.
43 Pauls D L, Towbin K E, Leckman J F, *et al.* Gilles de la Tourette's syndrome and obsessive compulsive disorder. *Arch Gen Psychiatry* 1986b;**43**:1180–1182.
44 Jenkins R L and Ashby H B. Gilles de la Tourette syndrome in identical twins. *Arch Neurology* 1983;**40**:249–251.
45 Rapoport J L. The neurology of obsessive-compulsive disorder. *J Am Med Assoc* 1988;**260**:2888–2890.
46 Behar D, Rapoport J L, Berg M A *et al.* Computerised tomography and neuro-psychological test measures in adolescents with obsessive-compulsive disorder. *Am J Psychiatry* 1984;**141**:363–369.
47 Garber H J, Ananth J V, Chiu L C *et al.* Nuclear magnetic resonance study of obsessive-compulsive disorder. *Am J Psychiatry* 1989;**146**:1001–1005.
48 Laplane D, Widlocher D, Pillon B *et al.* Compulsive behaviour of the obsessional type with bilateral circumscribed pallidostriatal necrosis (encephalopathy following a wasp sting). *Rev Neurol (Paris)* 1981;**137**:269–276.
49 Laplane D, Baulac M, Pillon B, *et al.* Perte de l'auto-activation psychique. Activite compulsive d'allure obsessionelle. Lesion lenticulaire bilaterale. *Rev Neurol (Paris)* 1982;**138**:137–141.
50 Swedo S E, Rapoport J L, Cheslow D L. High prevalence of obsessive-compulsive symptoms in patients with Sydenham's chorea. *Am J Psychiatry* 1989;**146**:246–249.
51 Luxenberg J S, Swedo S E, Flament M F *et al.* Neuroanatomical abnormalities in obsessive-compulsive disorder. *Am J Psychiatry* 1988;**145**:1089–1093.
52 Baxter L R, Phelps M E, Mazziotta J C *et al.* Local cerebral glucose metabolic rates in obsessive-compulsive disorder. A comparison with rates in unipolar depression and in normal controls. *Arch Gen Psychiatry* 1987;**44**:211–218.
53 Williams A C, Owen C and Heath D A. A compulsive movement disorder with cavitation of caudate nucleus. *J Neurol Neurosurg Psychiatry* 1988;**51**:447–448.
54 Pitman R K and Jenike M A. Coprolalia in obsessive-compulsive disorder: a missing link. *J Nerv Ment Dis* 1988;**176**:311–313.
55 Luxenberger H. Hereditat und Familientypus der Zwangsneurotiker. *Arch Psychiatr* 1930;**91**:590–594.
56 Lewis A. Problems of obsessional illness. *Proc Roy Soc Med* 1935;**29**:325–336.
57 Brown F W. Heredity in the psychoneuroses (summary). *Proc Roy Soc Med* 1942;**35**:785–790.

58 Kringlen E. Obsessional neurotics: a long term follow-up. *Br J Psychiatry* 1965;**111**: 709–722.
59 Rosenberg C M. Familial aspects of obsessional neurosis. *Br J Psychiatry* 1967; **113**:405–413.
60 Carey G. A Clinical Genetic Twin Study of Obsessional and Phobic States. PhD Thesis, University of Minnesota.
61 Insel T R, Hoover C and Murphy D L. Parents of patients with obsessive-compulsive disorder. *Psychol Med* 1983;**13**:807–811.
62 Rasmussen S A and Tsuang M T. Clinical characteristics and family history in DSMIII obsessive-compulsive disorder. *Am J Psychiatry* 1986;**143**:317–322.
63 Lenane M C, Swedo S E, Leonard H, Cheslow D L, Rapoport J L, Pauls D L. Obsessive compulsive disorder in first degree relatives of obsessive compulsive disorder children. *Proc Am Psychiatr Assoc*. Montreal, Canada. 1988.
64 Pauls D L, Raymond C L, Hurst C R, Rasmussen S, Goodman W and Leckman J F. Transmission of obsessive compulsive disorder and associated behaviours. *Proc Soc Biol Psychiatry*. Montreal, Canada. 1988.
65 Pitman R K. Pierre Janet on obsessive compulsive disorder (1903). *Arch Gen Psychiatry* 1987;**44**:226–232.

PSYCHOSURGERY IN OBSESSIONAL-COMPULSIVE DISORDER
Old Techniques and New Data

J M Bird and Carol D Crow

Burden Neurological Hospital, Bristol

OLD TECHNIQUES – AN HISTORICAL REVIEW

Early History

In 1867 Broca reported the finding by the American anthropologist E G Squier of a skull from the prehistoric period which had been dug up in Peru.[1] Over the vault there was a hole which was clearly man-made, Broca also observed signs of infection in the bone around the opening, suggesting that the patient had at least survived the operation. This then was evidence of a neurosurgical procedure being carried out in the prehistoric period. Since then several more such skulls have been found, particularly in Incan excavations. It is unclear why these operations were performed, but it has been shown that they were performed on skulls where there was evidence of brain disease, such as bony erosion.

The first modern account of psychosurgery was that of Burckhardt in 1891 from Switzerland.[2] He operated, rather haphazardly, to sever various connections in the brain in patients who were "incurably insane" – one died, one developed epilepsy, one improved and four others showed no change. For a definition of psychosurgery see Figure 1.

Figure 1.

PSYCHOSURGERY

Definition: 1) A surgical intervention
– to sever, remove, destroy or stimulate brain tissue

2) With the intent of modifying disturbances of behaviour, thought or mood

3) For which no organic pathological cause can be demonstrated

Problems with this – does it include surgery for pain and epilepsy?

During the latter half of the 19th century, and the first 30 years of this century, animal work was carried out, particularly by the British Neurologist, Sir David Ferrier,[3] into the effects of damage to the frontal lobes of monkeys. This work grew from the case of Phineas Gage, a construction foreman, who had had a tamping iron (3'7" long) blasted through his brain. He recovered almost immediately and was able to speak. However, his personality showed marked changes. He became "irreverent", childish, profane, impatient and capricious, so that friends said he was "no longer Gage". He died 12½ years after the accident and his story was published by Harlow in 1848. Ferrier considered that this indicated a vital role for the frontal lobes in the maintainance of personality.[3]

In 1886, Ferrier[3] wrote that if the frontal lobes of monkeys were destroyed they became tamer and more docile. Following from this, Fulton and Jacobsen carried out a series of experiments in which selective lesions were made in the frontal lobes of chimpanzees. In particular they described the effects of an operation on Becky, a previously violent chimp, who became much gentler – in 1935 they wrote "It was as if the animal had joined the happiness cult of Elder Michaeux" and "had placed its burdens on the Lord".[4]

Human Psychosurgery – Pioneering days

When Jacobsen presented this work in London, present in the audience was the 61 year old Professor of Neurology at Lisbon, Egas Moniz. (Prof. Moniz

Fig 2

HISTORY I – PIONEERING DAYS

BURCKHARDT 1891[2] (Switzerland)	– The first psychosurgery
HARLOW 1861[29]	– The case of Phineas Gage
FERRIER 1886[3]	– Ablation of frontal lobes of monkeys
FULTON & JACOBSEN 1920s[4]	– Experiments on frontal lobes of chimps. Particularly "Becky"
MONIZ[5] (& LIMA) 1935	– Alcohol injection in 20 psychiatric patients
FREEMAN & WATTS[7] 1940s – 50s	– Standard leucotomy (40-50,000 performed in US by 1971 12,000 performed in UK by 1954) – Also Radical Leucotomy, Transorbital Leucotomy

had previously been Portugal's foreign minister and had also invented the cerebral angiogram). Moniz had, for some time, been speculating about the possibility of carrying out neurosurgical operations for the relief of mental disorders. Fulton and Jacobsen's work seems to have crystallized his ideas. In November 1935, under Moniz' instruction, the surgeon Lund injected alcohol to destroy the white matter of the frontal lobes in 20 patients – all survived, 7 recovered completely and 7 were somewhat improved. In 1949 Moniz was awarded the Nobel prize for his work on leucotomy.[5]

Freeman (a psychiatrist) and Watts (a neurosurgeon) – from Washington, took up the work.[6] They modified Moniz' operation in various ways and by 1971, 40-50,000 operations had been done in the US (and by 1954, 12,000 in the UK). Freeman had personally been involved in 3,500 operations. However, in the late 1960s the numbers started dropping dramatically; by 1977 only 250 per year were done in the UK and by 1981 only 70.

During the heyday, a variety of techniques and instruments were used; operations usually involved cutting of various kinds (leucotomes of varying ingenuity and elegance were invented).[7] The first British leucotomy was performed in 1941 by Mr. Wilway at the Burden Neurological Institute.

A More Scientific Approach

In the late 1960s, because of an increase in understanding of the functions and connections of the frontal lobes, a more "scientific" psychosurgery emerged. This involved the use of much more circumscribed lesions and a much more careful choice of patients. An understanding of the fronto-limbic connections and of the importance of these to emotional, rather than thought disorders, led to a concentration on the treatment of intractable mood and neurotic disorders rather than schizophrenia. It also led to operating on limbic structures as well as the frontal lobes.

Fig 3

HISTORY II – A MORE SCIENTIFIC APPROACH

SPIEGEL 1947[10] – Stereotaxis
WARD 1948[9] – Cingulotomy
KNIGHT 1960s[11] – Stereotatic Sub caudate Tractotomy
KELLY 1960s[25] – Stereotactic Limbic Leucotomy
CROW 1960s[21] – Multifocal Leucocoagulation (Orbital frontal ± paracingulate)
HITCHCOCK & CAIRNS[30] 1960s – Amygdalotomy

1977 250 operations per year in UK
1981 70 operations per year in UK

The functions of the cingulate gyrus became an important aspect in the understanding of emotional disorders, as well as other aspects of the "circuit of emotion", described by Papez.[8] In 1948 Ward carried out the first cingulotomy on humans and since then this has become an important aspect of psychosurgery.[9] The amygdala was operated on since it was found that amygdalotomy in rats led to them becoming docile.

84

In 1947 Spiegel invented the stereotactic apparatus, versions of which have since been widely used in all precision neurosurgery.[10] This allowed the placement, by various means, of much more precise lesions. In addition to injecting and cutting, the lesions have been produced by inserting seeds of radioactive Ytrium (Y90),[11] by freezing (using cryosurgery – inserting a cooling cannula and injecting liquid nitrogen). Electrically induced heat, has also been used since the 1950s. This is the technique of "thermocoagulation" in which an electrical current is passed through the free end of an electrode needle.

A variety of operation sites have been used but most have tended to centre on the orbital white matter of the frontal cortex and the cingulate or paracingulate white matter. (Fig 4).

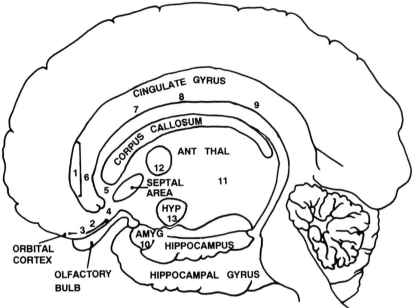

Frontal Lobe Procedures
1 Bimedial leucotomy
2 Yttrium lesions in subcortical white matter
3 Orbital undercutting
4 Basal tractotomy and substantia innominotomy
5 Anterior capsulotomy (destruction of fibres of internal capsule)
6 Mesioleviotomy (similar to rostral cingulotomy but lesion invades geny "knee" of corpus callosum)

Cingulotomies
7 Anterior cingulotomy

8 Mid-cingulotomy
9 Posterior cingulotomy

Amygdalectomy
10 Amygdalectomy or amygdalotomy

Thalatomies
11 Dorsomedial, centromedian, parafascicula muclei
12 Anterior thalatomy

Hypothalotomy
13 Posterior, ventromedial and lateral hypothalamic targets

Diagram of the various psychosurgical procedures[13]
Courtesy of ELLIOT S VALENSTEIN
Reproduced by kind permission of the author

EVALUATION OF PROCEDURES

There have been many thousands of articles written about psychosurgery. By 1964 at least 4000 had been published, but as a review of that time said "a ridiculously small number have paid even lip service to experimental design".[12] In 1977 the Royal College of Psychiatrists proposed a prospective controlled trial of neurosurgery, but sadly this was never started. Of course, by 1981 only 70 operations per year were being carried out, so perhaps it was unnecessary. On the other hand we may be missing a potentially very effective treatment which has fallen into misuse because of misunderstanding.

Fig 5.

EVALUATION

By 1964 – 4,000 papers

   1961 – Tooth & Brook[14] (M O H)

   1975 – Stone[15]

   1977 – Valenstein[13] (US Commission)

      – 90% of papers were of low scientific value

   1982 – O'Callaghan & Carroll[16] – "no scientific decision can be made"

But – recent improvements:

1) Neurosurgical techniques more precise

2) Anatomy and physiology better understood

3) Diagnostic accuracy much improved

4) Improved consensus on which patients to treat with psychosurgery

Conclusion:	*Operations:*	Cingulectomy
		Orbital Frontal Leucotomy
	Disorders:	Obsessional Compulsive Disorder
		also Anxiety Disorders
		Depressive Disorders

In 1977 Valenstein was asked by a US National Commission to survey all the recent studies. He found that 90% of the studies published between 1970 and 1976 were of low or very low scientific value.[13] This conclusion was based on a previously agreed scale for assessing the scientific basis of therapeutic studies. Other reviews have included a British one supported by the Ministry of Health,[14] and a USA group, called The Massachussetts Task Force on Psychosurgery.[15] Again, both were unable to come to any firm conclusions on the efficacy of psychosurgery because of the sorry state of the literature.

In 1982 O'Callaghan and Carroll published the latest such broad based review, but were unable to come to any firm scientific decision.[16] However they were able to draw up some guidelines based on the published studies. They felt that there have been recent improvements. Neurosurgical technique is now much more precise and accurate, there has been an improved understanding of the anatomy and physiology of the regions concerned. In addition diagnostic accuracy in psychiatry has improved and there has been an increased consensus about which forms of disorder are best treated in this way. It must always be remembered that neurosurgery is used as a last resort in most cases. Whether this is as it shold be or not can be debated.

Their conclusions are that *cingulectomy* and perhaps *orbital frontal leucotomy* are useful procedures, giving significantly better than expected recovery rates.

As far as the disorders best treated by neurosurgery are concerned, only obsessional disorder consistently scores highly. Anxiety disorders and chronic depressive disorders score less highly. For a summary of published results see Fig 6.

Fig 6

DISORDERS – RESULTS OF SURGERY

Obsessional – Compulsive Neurosis
65% improved or greatly improved with cingulotomy + bifrontal operations (only 50% with bifrontal alone).[25,26]

Anxiety
58% improved or greatly, improved with bifrontal alone.[24,27]

Unipolar Depression
68% improved with bifrontal alone.[24,27]

Bipolar Depression
Substantial improvement in 5 out of 9 patients.[31]

Violent Behaviour
Case reports of improvements following amygdalectomy.[30]

Schizophrenia
Extensively used at first, but *not* recently. Kelly[32] – 19 patients with high anxiety, depression or obsessional-compulsive symptoms. 12 were improved or much improved.

It must of course be remembered that all these results are in open studies of uncontrolled groups. However, it must also be noted that *all* the patients reported upon had previously suffered many years of intractable illness, unresponsive to other treatments and that the prognosis for natural recovery in such cases, especially of obsessional compulsive disorder, is very poor.[17]

87

ADVERSE EFFECTS

It is well known that the early and extensive leucotomies and lobotomies caused major personality changes. The first description in the UK of such adverse effects was reported from the Burden Neurological Institute[18] and resulted in the cessation of such operations there until the most careful and painstaking of psychosurgical procedures, multifocal leucocoagulation, was developed by Crow *et al* in the late 1950s.[19]

Contrary to the early procedures, modern techniques result in few if any, adverse effects. Mortality now approaches zero. There is a 1-2% risk of development of epilepsy, usually very easily controlled. In about 5-10% subtle personality changes may be detected, usually with some reduction in drive and sometimes with a degree of social disinhibition. Cognitive deficits are not detectable, indeed at times a degree of apparent improvement in cognitive abilities has been demonstrated, probably due to an improved ability to concentrate. A worsening of addictive or suicidal behaviour has on occasion been shown if it was present pre-operatively, but not otherwise. Such behaviour may be a relative contra-indication.

ADDITIONAL CONSIDERATIONS

Other important considerations, not discussed extensively here, include the ethics of the procedure and the need for fully informed consent and for discussion with the patient and family. The legal requirements of the Mental Health Act are extensive. Public and psychiatric attitudes to the procedure have probably had a major effect on its usage as well as advances in other forms of management. It is clear that not only must all patients have undergone an exhaustive course of Behaviour Therapy before operation is considered, but that Behaviour Therapy must be continued after the operation. Indeed we would suggest that one of the main effects of the operation is to enable the patient to respond to Behaviour Therapy. It is our firm opinion that careful preparation of the patient and continued behavioural psychotherapy and support post-operatively are vital to success. It has also been the impression of the team at the Burden Neurological Institute that better results are achieved if the disorder appears to be "constitutional" in the sense of existing as part of the personality from an early age, if the individual is naturally truthful and if there is a supportive family. (Fig 7).

Fig 7
INDICATIONS FOR PSYCHOSURGERY

1. Non-psychotic, informal, capable of giving fully informed consent.
2. Suffering from: Anxiety Neurosis
   Obsessional Compulsive Neurosis
   Depressive illness
3. Chronic, unremitting illness for at least 2 years with severe lilfe-disruption
4. Failure to respond to all recognised forms of therapy (physical *and* psychological)
5. Absence of major addictive behaviour
6. Better results if: "constitutional" disorder
   truthful
   supportive family

MULTIFOCAL LEUCOCOAGULATION

During the late 1950s, H J Crow (Neuropsychiatrist), R Cooper (Scientist) and D G Phillips (Neurosurgeon) developed a procedure involving the implantation of 10-20 sheaves of gold wires (containing up to 72 electrodes)into the orbital and paracingulate regions of the frontal lobes by stereotactic technique.[19,20,21] Once implanted the wires were left *in situ* for up to 10 months. Individual electrode sites were identified as being in white or grey matter using electrical stimulation; grey matter produces a characteristic after-discharge and such sites can be avoided when coagulating. Over the ensuing weeks or months reversible "polarisation" and subsequently irreversible electro-coagulation can be carried out little by little and progressively.[22] Progress in relieving symptoms and any emergence of adverse side effects can be closely monitored and the degree of white matter destruction tailored to each patient.[23]

Results

The most extensive follow-up of any group of psychosurgery patients was carried out by Crow C D. This is the first publication of those results. In all, 142 patients were operated on between 1960 and 1974. 105 were interviewed at a mean of 12 year follow up, and reliable information obtained on a further 23. The mean length of pre-operative illness was 9.3 years. 84 of the patients suffered from obsessional compulsive disorder (OCD), the others from anxiety disorder. Operative mortality was nil, operative morbidity minimal (one patient had a transient monoplegia, six showed brief meningeal irritation). One patient without previous leucotomy developed epilepsy which was entirely controlled with an anticonvulsant.

Two of the 90 OCD patients developed a severe personality change almost certainly not due to the procedure – one subsequent to a massive overdose and one due to development of a late dementing illness. Four patients showed moderate change, three with a decrease in drive and one with mild social disinhibition. Six patients showed minimal personality change, often regarded as positive by relatives (such as being less withdrawn, more outspoken). It is important to note that 85% showed no personality change detectable to themselves, relatives, general practitioner or (if still relevant) psychiatrist. No patient showed reduction in WAIS score (apart from the two with severe non-related changes) and in fact a mean increase was shown from 105 to 113.

Overall results are shown in Table 1. It can be seen that 68% were either completely recovered or had mild symptoms which did not interfere with their lives. More than half (56%) of males and 27% of females, were now in full-time employment (cf. 0% pre-operatively). 80% of females had a normal capacity for housework. There were, at follow up, 54% of patients on no psychotropic drugs and 59% not receiving any psychiatric care. Creative ability was often enhanced and patients had written books of poetry and short stories, obtained Degrees, undertaken scientific research work, and one patient had taken up work as a doctor again.

Table 1

MULTIFOCAL LEUCOCAGULATION
OVERALL RESULTS

%

Global Assessment[24]

I	Recovered, no symptoms, no treatment required	30	
II	Well, mild residual symptoms, no interferences with life	38	} 68%
III	Improved, but still significant interfering symptoms	26	
IV	Unchanged	6	
V	Worse	0	

NB Concordance between BNI assessors and current medical attendants   85%

Concordance between BNI assessors and patients and relatives   83%

Relapses of OCD had occurerd in 21%, but 89% of these had shown complete recovery, with relapses lasting less than a month in 79%.

In fact relapse was very rare unless recurrent depression was also present and pre-existing severe depression indicated a less successful outcome. A summary of outcome results is presented in Table 2.

Table 2

MULTIFOCAL LEUCOCOAGULATION
SUMMARY OF RESULTS (in OCD)

No operative morbidity of more than a few days
Post-operative epilepsy in 1 case out of 128
No detectable personality change in 85%
Increase in IQ by 8 points
Complete or almost complete recovery in 68%
Importance of continuing behaviour therapy and after care

SUMMARY

Psychosurgical procedures, after gross over-use which brought them into understandable and, often, well deserved disrepute, emerged in the 1960s as more carefully considered therapeutic endeavours. However a natural repugnance (though often unthinking, and more on the part of therapist than patient), combined with the impossibility of carrying out double-blind controlled trials, has led to the near disappearance of psycho-surgical activity. The extensive follow-up study reported here, as well as those reported elsewhere,[24-28] suggests that precise psychosurgical operations may be indicated in severe, unremitting OCD when all other treatments have failed. In such cases about two thirds will recover completely, or almost completely, and impossible though it may seem to some, there are negligible, if any, adverse effects.

REFERENCES

1 Broca P. *Cas singulier de trepanation chez les Incas. Bull Soc Anthropol* 1967;**2**:403–408.

2 Burckhardt G. *Ueber Rinden excisioner, als Beitrag zur operativen therapie der Psycochosen. Allg Z Psychiatrie* 1891;**47**:463–548.

3 Ferrier D. The Functions of the Brain 2ndEd (London:Smith,Elder). 1886.

4 Hutton E L, Fleming G W T H and Fox F C. Early results of prefrontal leucotomy. *Lancet* 1941;**2**:3–7.

5 Moniz E. How I succeeded in performing the prefrontal leukotomy. In: Sackler A *et al* eds. The Great Psychodynamic Therapies in psychiatry. (New York, Harper & Row). 1956.

6 Freeman W and Watts J W. Psychosurgery. (Springfield Il Charles C Thomas). 1942.

7 Freeman W and Watts J W. Psychosurgery 2ndEd (Springfield Il Charles C Thomas). 1950.

8 Papex J W. A proposed mechanism of emotion. *Arch Neurol Psychiatry* 1937;**38**:725–743.

9 Ward A A Jr. The anterior cingulate gyrus and personality. *Res Publ Assoc Neurol Ment Dis* 1948;**47**:419–420.

10 Spiegel E A, Wycis H T, Marks M and Lee A J. Stereotaxic apparatus for operations on the human brain. *Science* 1947;**106**;349–530.

11 Knight G G. Stereotactic tractotomy in the surgical treatment of mental illness. *J Neurol, Neurosurg, Psychiatry* 1965;**28**:304–310.

12 Canadian Medical Association Journal. Standard lobotomy: The end of an era. *Canad Med Assoc J* 1964;**91**:1228–1229.

13 Valenstein E S. The practice of psychosurgery : A survey of the literature (1971-1976). (Washington, US Dept Health, Education and Welfare). 1977.

14 Tooth G C and Newton M P. Leucotomy in England and Wales (1942-1954). Ministry of Health report No 104. (London : HMSO). 1961.

15 Stone A A. Psychosurgery in Massachusetts : A task force report. *Mass J Ment HealthO'Callaghan M A J and Carroll D. Psychosurgery : A scientific analysis (Lancaster, MTP Press). 1982.*

17 Bebbington P. *The prevalence of obsessive compulsive disorder within the community. This volume.*

18 Hutton E L, Fleming G W T H and Fox F C. *Early results of prefrontal leucotomy. Lancet* 1941;**2**:3–7.

19 Crow H J, Cooper R and Phillips D G. Controlled multifocal frontal leucotomy for psychiatric illness. *J Neurol, Neurosurg, Psychiat* 1961;**24**:343–360.

20 Crow H J, Cooper R and Phillips D G. Progressive Leucotomy. In Masserman J H (ed) Current Psychiatric Therapies Vol III. (New York: Grune and Stratton). 1963.

21 Crow H J. Intracerebral polarisation and multifocal leucocoagulation in some psychiatric illnesses. *Psychiatr Neurol Neurochirurg* 1973;**76**:365–381.

22 Crow H J and Cooper R. Stimulation, polarisation and coagulation using intracerebral implanted electrodes during the investigation and treatment of psychiatric and other disorders. *Med Prog Technol* 1972;**1**:92–102.

23 Crow H J. The treatment of anxiety and obsessionality with chronically implanted electrodes. In Smith J S, and Kiloh L G (eds) Psychosurgery and Society (Oxford:Pergamon). 1977.

24 Bridges P K, Goktepe E O and Maratos J. A comparative review of patients with obsessional illness and with depression treated by psychosurgery. *Br J Psychiatry* 1973;**123**:663–674.

25 Kelly D, Richardson A, Mitchell-Heggs N, Greenup J, Chen and Hafner R J. Stereotactic limbic leucotomy : A preliminary report on 40 patients. *Br J Psychiatry* 1973;**123**:141–148.

26 Knight G G. Further observations from an experience of 660 cases of stereotactic tractotomy. *Postgrad Med J* 1973;**49**:845–854.

27 Goktepe C O, Young L B and Bridges P K. A further review of the results of stereotactic subcaudate tractotomy. *Br J Psychiatry* 1975;**126**;270–280.

28 Ballantine H T, Levy B S, Dagi T F and Giriunas I B. Cingulotomy for psychiatric illness: Report of 13 years experience. In: Sweet W H *et al* eds. Neurosurgical treatment in Psychiatry, Pain and Epilepsy (Baltimore, University Park Press). 1977.

29 Harlow J M. Passage of an iron through the head. *Boston Med Surg J* 1848;**39**:389–393.

30 Hitchcock E and Cairns U. Amygdalectomy. *Postgrad Med J* 1973;**49**:894–904.

31 Poynton A, Bridges P K and Bartlett J R. Resistant Bipolar Affective Disorder treated by stereotactic subcaudate tractotomy. *Br J Psychiatry* 1988;**152**:354–358.

32 Kelly D. Anxiety and Emotions – Physiological basis and treatment. Springfield Il, Charles C Thomas). 1980.

LIST OF DELEGATES
OBSESSIVE COMPULSIVE DISORDER SYMPOSIUM
Friday 6th April 1990

Mrs R M J Ablett
Stockton-on-Tees

Dr W D Addis
Co Antrim

Dr N Ahmed
South Shields

Ms I Ahuja
Hitchin

Dr M J Akhtar
South Shields

Dr D S Allen
Reading

Dr J M Alvarez-Ude
Haywards Heath

Dr J B Anderson
London

Dr A Ansfield
London

Dr R A Baker
Southampton

Dr Balakrishnan
Ipswich

Dr D Baldwin
London

Ms R Barber
Basingstoke

Dr R K Baruah
Nottingham

Dr R E Bates
Farnborough

Dr G Beaumont
Stockport

Dr I Berg
Leeds

Dr B R Bhadrinath
Chatham

Dr A Bhattacharyya
Wellingborough

Dr R Bhuvanendran
Brentwood

Dr J Bird
London

Dr A Bond
London

Dr J A Boodhoo
Solihull

Dr O Bowey
Epsom

Dr C Bowler
Etwall

Miss A Bryan
Newbury

Dr R Buller
Germany

Dr H P Burrowes
Leeds

Miss M Byrne
London

Mr D Callinan
Buckingham

Dr L S Cantlay
Cleveland

Dr R J Carlson
London

Mr J Carreira
Ashford

Dr J Carvalhinho
King's Lynn

Dr B C Chaparala
Scunthorpe

Dr P Chapman
Bristol

Dr T Chein
Salisbury

Ms K E Cheshire
Edinburgh

Dr I D Chisholm
Bristol

Mr N Clarke
Beckenham

Dr A M Cobb
Cheanley

Dr J P Cobb
London

Dr J J Cockburn
Epsom

Ms L J Colson
London

Dr J R Compton
Fareham

Dr W P Conlon
Dudley

Dr C G Conway
Ivybridge

Mr R Cook
Leicester

Dr F Cosgrove
Trowbridge

Dr V Crawford
London

Dr D P Cronin
Brentwood

Dr D C Crow
Bristol

Mrs S J Crowley
Norwich

Dr J Dark
London

Mr S Darnley
Maidstone

Mr A Dassrath
London

Dr M Davys
London

Ms J L Dawkins
London

Miss R Day
Beckenham

Ms A Deale
London

Dr J Deans
Carmarthen

Miss L D Denford
London

Dr M Denham
Essex

Dr V De Silva
Colchester

Dr H E De Waal
Wirral

Dr M Dhadphale
London

Dr L Dratcu
London

Dr F J Dunne
Brentwood

Col. H Ferguson
Northampton

Mr H Fisher
Manchester

Mrs J C Fordy
Edgbaston

Dr M F Foyle
London

Dr R France
Camberley

Dr O S Frank
London

Ms L Franklin
Hitchin

Dr C Friedman
London

Dr T Galla
Newcastle

Dr G R Gallimore
Dorchester

Dr N Gene-Cos
London

Dr S K Ghosh
Hereford

Ms M Gibson
Epsom

Dr M J Gleeson
London

Dr P Goodyear
Birmingham

Dr A M Grape
Brecon

Mr M Greener
London

Dr M Gunaratnam
Darlington

Dr K M Hadi
Stevenage

Dr S Haque
Harlow

Miss P J Harries
Poole

Dr N J Hart
Camberley

Dr B K W Ho
Watford

Mr M Hunt
London

Ms B Hunter
London

Dr E M Irwin
Birmingham

Dr G Ivbijaro
Derby

Dr V S Iyer
Hull

94

Mr I Jackes
Surbiton

Dr D Jadresic
London

Dr M Jasen
Radlett

Dr N Jeganathan
Derby

Dr S Jogees
Ispwich

Dr A Jones
Oxford

Dr S B Jones
Wallingford

Dr G Kanakaratnam
Hitchin

Dr R Kandavel
Coulsdon

Dr L G H Karunapala
Brentwood

Dr A W Katz
London

Dr L Katzenell
St Albans

Dr D Kelly
London

Dr F J Kelly
London

Dr M I Khalid
St Albans

Dr T G Kidd
Chertsey

Dr N I Kitson
London

Dr J van der Knaap
London

Dr B W Knights
Norwich

Dr Y Kon
Medway

Dr M J Kosler
Carshalton

Dr M Kularatna
Wickford

Dr E Kupusmitt
Edgware

Dr S Lack
London

Dr T Lambert
London

Dr F Lappin
Stevenage

Mr M J Latham
London

Dr A R Lillywhite
Devizes

Dr L E C Lim
Kingston-upon-Thames

Dr M Livingston
Glasgow

Dr A Lowe
Worcester

Mr S McAfee
Liverpool

Ms F McClaren
Windlesham

Dr J L McClure
Welwyn Garden City

Dr C McDonald
Warlingham

Ms T McGoldrick
Bridge of Allan

Ms A McGowan
London

Dr A A McKirdy
Lindfield

Dr H R Markar
Ipswich

Dr P H Mars
Abergavenny

DR Mawalagedera
Epsom

Mr J Mercer
Cambridge

Dr W I Mikhail
Dartford

Dr R G Millward
Crewe

Dr V N Minas
Wickford

Dr H Molony
Teddington

Dr D Montgomery
London

Mr B Morrissey
Coventry

Dr S Morten
London

Dr S Moser
Woodbridge

Dr M S Muir
Ely

Ms I Murphy
Hitchin

Dr I K Mutiboko
St Leonards

Dr Muttunayagam
Chertsey

Dr V A G Nanayakkara
St Albans

Dr M E N Naquib
Epsom

Dr T U K Nasir
Bradford

Mr C Nethercott
Weymouth

Mr H I Noshirvani
London

Dr P Nott
Southampton

Dr T J O'Grady
Lincoln

Mr J O'Neill-Byrne
London

Dr R B F Orr
Newton Abbot

Mr M O'Sullivan
Warwick

Mrs M Outschoorn
London

Mr S Palanisamy
London

Dr A H Parvis
London

Dr G H Patel
Brentwood

Ms P Pattman
Nottingham

Dr A Perez
Northampton

Dr L Pilowsky
London

Dr S M Ponnappa
Staines

Dr W B F Prothero
Ashford

Dr S Rabee
Chertsey

Dr M Ramgoolam
Cardiff

Dr J Rao
Bedford

Dr B K Rathod
Leigh

Dr A Regan
Watford

Mr S Regel
Nottingham

Dr E H Reid
Dundee

Dr A Rhys
Dyfed

Mr P Rice
Brentwood

Baroness von Richthofen
London

Ms S von Richthofen
London

Mrs B Rickinson
Edgbaston

Dr H Ring
London

Mr N Riordon
London

Dr P H Rogers
Northampton

Dr G Rooney
London

Ms G Rowley
Epsom

Dr S R Sadik
Maidstone

Dr B N Saha
Esher

Ms J Salter
Wallingford

Dr Samarasinghe
Welwyn

Dr G Samuel
Windlesham

Mrs S E Saunders
Buckingham

Dr D H Seijas
London

Dr S A Selim
Blackburn

Dr S Shakespear
Colchester

Dr Shanmuganathan
Dartford

Dr A Sharratt
London

Dr C R Shawcross
Fareham

Dr J Short
Bristol

Dr A M Siddiqui
Londonderry

Dr W R Silveira
Coventry

Dr J C Silveria
London

Dr D Singh
Blackburn

Dr A Smirnov
Oxford

Dr E B O Smith
Oxford

Dr L Steen
Prestwich

Ms L J Steen
Rochdale

Dr D Steinberg
Beckenham

Ms M H Stones
High Wycombe

Dr C L Taylor
Cumbria

Dr Tay Woo Kheng
London

Ms D Thapinta
Milton Keynes

Dr K Thinn
Birmingham

Dr S Thomas
London

Dr F Toates
Milton Keynes

Dr F Tylden
London

Mrs M A Vining
Surbiton

Dr J D Waldman
London

Mrs K Waters
Norwich

Dr V A Watkin
Barnet

Mrs A Watts
Weymouth

Mrs P Westcott
London

Dr B K Wharton
Northampton

Miss F A White
St Albans

Mr G M Whitford
Alton

Dr S C Will
Inverness

Mr M Williams
London

Mrs M Williamson
Weymouth

Ms J Yakeley
London

Dr E H Zaghloul
Burton-on-Trent

Dr K M Zaw
Gloucester

MEDICAL RELATIONS PUBLICATIONS

CURRENT APPROACHES SERIES

Bulimia Nervosa   (reprint April 1990)
Endometrial Carcinoma
Risk/Benefits of Antidepressants
Childbirth as a Life Event
Sleep Disorders
Advances in Pancreatitis
Sudden Cardiac Death
Neuropsychiatric Aspects of AIDS
The Problem of Recurrent Abdominal Pain
Breaking Bad News
Mental Retardation
Panic – Symptom or Disorder?
Modern Trends in Aetiology and Management of CIN
Colorectal Cancer

The above publications can be obtained by writing to:-
DUPHAR MEDICAL RELATIONS
Duphar Laboratories Limited
West End
Southampton
SO3 3JD